T0259375

Pediatric Ultrasound Part 2

Guest Editor

BRIAN D. COLEY, MD

ULTRASOUND CLINICS

www.ultrasound.theclinics.com

January 2010 • Volume 5 • Number 1

SAUNDERS an imprint of ELSEVIER, Inc.

W.B. SAUNDERS COMPANY
A Division of Elsevier Inc.

1600 John F. Kennedy Boulevard • Suite 1800 • Philadelphia, Pennsylvania 19103-2899

http://www.theclinics.com

ULTRASOUND CLINICS Volume 5, Number 1
January 2010 ISSN 1556-858X, ISBN-13: 978-1-4377-1945-1

Editor: Barton Dudlick
Developmental Editor: Theresa Collier

Ultrasound Clinics (ISSN 1556-858X) is published quarterly by W.B. Saunders, 360 Park Avenue South, New York, NY 10010-1710. Months of publication are January, April, July, and October. Business and editorial offices: 1600 John F. Kennedy Boulevard, Suite 1800, Philadelphia, Pennsylvania 19103-2899. Accounting and circulation offices: 6277 Sea Harbor Drive, Orlando, FL 32887-4800. Periodicals postage paid at New York, NY, and additional mailing offices. Subscription prices are $204 per year for (US individuals), $279 per year for (US institutions), $102 per year for (US students and residents), $232 per year for (Canadian individuals), $312 per year for (Canadian institutions), $247 per year for (international individuals), $312 per year for (international institutions), and $123 per year for (Canadian and foreign students/residents). To receive student/resident rate, orders must be accompanied by name of affiliated institution, date of term, and the signature of program/residency coordinator on institution letterhead. Orders will be billed at individual rate until proof of status is received. Foreign air speed delivery is included in all Clinics subscription prices. All prices are subject to change without notice. **POSTMASTER:** Send address changes to *Ultrasound Clinics,* Elsevier Health Sciences Division, Subscription Customer Service, 3251 Riverport Lane, Maryland Heights, MO 63043. **Customer Service (orders, claims, online, change of address): Telephone: 1-800-654-2452 (U.S. and Canada); 314-447-8871(outside U.S. and Canada). Fax: 314-447-8029. E-mail: journalscustomerservice-usa@elsevier.com (for print support); journalsonlinesupport-usa@elsevier.com (for online support).**

Reprints: For copies of 100 or more, of articles in this publication, please contact the Commercial Reprints Department, Elsevier Inc., 360 Park Avenue South, New York, NY 10010-1710. Tel.: (+1) 212-633-3812; Fax: (+1) 212-462-1935; E-mail: reprints@elsevier.com.

Contributors

GUEST EDITOR

BRIAN D. COLEY, MD
Department of Radiology, Nationwide
Children's Hospital, Columbus, Ohio; Clinical
Professor of Radiology and Pediatrics, The
Ohio State University College of Medicine
and Public Health, Columbus, Ohio

AUTHORS

RICHARD D. BELLAH, MD
Associate Professor of Radiology and
Pediatrics, University of Pennsylvania School
of Medicine; Director, Division of Ultrasound,
The Children's Hospital of Philadelphia,
Philadelphia, Pennsylvania

THOMAS P. BOULDEN, MD
Professor, Department of Radiology, University
of Tennessee Health Science Center;
LeBonheur Children's Medical Center,
Memphis, Tennessee

MICHEL CLAUDON, MD
Professor of Radiology, University of Nancy;
Department of Radiology, Children's Hospital,
Vandoeuvre les Nancy, France

HARRIS L. COHEN, MD, FACR
Chairman, Department of Radiology, University
of Tennessee Health Science Center; Medical
Director, Department of Radiology, LeBonheur
Children's Medical Center; Professor of
Radiology, Pediatrics and Obstetrics
and Gynecology, Memphis,
Tennessee

KASSA DARGE, MD, PhD
Professor of Radiology, University of
Pennsylvania School of Medicine; Chief,
Division of Body Imaging, The Children's
Hospital of Philadelphia, Philadelphia,
Pennsylvania

DANA DUMITRIU, MD
Department of Radiology, Children's Hospital,
Vandoeuvre les Nancy, France

MONICA S. EPELMAN, MD
Assistant Professor of Radiology, University
of Pennsylvania School of Medicine,
The Children's Hospital of Philadelphia,
Philadelphia, Pennsylvania

MARIE-AGNÈS GALLOY, MD
Department of Radiology, Children's Hospital,
Vandoeuvre les Nancy, France

LAURENT GAREL, MD
Clinical Professor of Radiology, Department
of Radiology, Radio-oncology and Nuclear
Medicine, University of Montreal; Radiologist,
Department of Medical Imaging,
Sainte-Justine Mother and Child University
Hospital Center, Montreal, Quebec, Canada

ELTON B. GREENE, MD
Resident, Department of Radiology, University
of Tennessee, Methodist University Hospital
Program, Memphis, Tennessee

JEANNE G. HILL, MD
Associate Professor of Radiology
and Pediatrics, Department of Radiology
and Radiological Science, Medical
University of South Carolina, Charleston,
South Carolina

BOAZ KARMAZYN, MD
Associate Professor of Radiology, Department of Pediatric Radiology, Riley Hospital for Children, Indiana University School of Medicine, Indianapolis, Indiana

KATHLEEN M. McCARTEN, MD, FACR
Associate Professor of Diagnostic Imaging and Pediatrics (Clinical), Department of Radiology, The Warren Alpert Medical School of Brown University; Radiologist, Rhode Island Hospital, Providence, Rhode Island

MARTHE M. MUNDEN, MD
Pediatric Radiology Department, Children's Health System of Alabama, Alabama Children's Hospital, Birmingham, Alabama; Currently Attending Radiologist at Singleton Associates, Edward B. Singleton Department of Diagnostic Imaging, Texas Children's Hospital, Houston, Texas

LAURA VARICH, MD
Pediatric Radiologist, Florida Hospital for Children, Orlando, Florida; Stanford University Medical Center, Stanford, California

Contents

In the past decade, the imaging approach to pediatric urinary tract infection (UTI) has been challenged by evidence-based literature and physician experience. The routine use of ultrasound (US) for first time uncomplicated pediatric UTI evaluation has become somewhat controversial as several studies have shown that US provides low yield for additional clinically useful information. Nevertheless, for all of its advantages, including its use for depicting structural urinary tract abnormalities, many pediatric practioners continue to include US as an integral part of their routine evaluation of first-time UTI in pediatric patients.

Cystic renal disease in children is subdivided into hereditary disorders and nongenetic conditions. Ultrasound is the cornerstone of imaging. In association with the family history, associated clinical features, and laboratory data, ultrasound allows a precise diagnosis in most instances. Prenatal imaging and postnatal correlations have been very contributive in outlining the natural history of cystic renal diseases in the pediatric age group.

Scrotal ultrasound (US) is the first, and usually only, imaging study for evaluation of scrotal pathologies. In many cases, scrotal US can provide a specific diagnosis. In other cases, US helps direct appropriate management. US is readily available with no need for any preparation or sedation. Therefore, it is used in urgent situations, such as acute scrotal pain, to aid in the diagnosis of testicular torsion. In boys with a scrotal mass, US helps differentiate between intratesticular and extratesticular tumors and pathologies that mimic scrotal tumors. US is used in evaluation of cryptorchidism, hydrocele, scrotal hernia, varicocele, and follow-up of testicular microlithiasis.

Ultrasound may be used as an alternative to radiography in evaluating the upper gastrointestinal tract of newborns and small infants due to proximity of the structures to the anterior abdominal wall and the ability to distend with fluid. Survival has increased significantly in very small premature infants resulting in a population that is fragile and vulnerable to external stresses. The gastrointestinal tract is at risk; ultrasound is the most noninvasive modality for evaluation and with Doppler has become the most predictive means of establishing bowel viability.

Ultrasound Clinics

THE CLINICS ARE NOW AVAILABLE ONLINE!

Access your subscription at:
www.theclinics.com

GOAL STATEMENT

The goal of the *Ultrasound Clinics* is to keep practicing radiologists and radiology residents up to date with current clinical practice in ultrasound by providing timely articles reviewing the state of the art in patient care.

ACCREDITATION

The *Ultrasound Clinics* is planned and implemented in accordance with the Essential Areas and Policies of the Accreditation Council for Continuing Medical Education (ACCME) through the joint sponsorship of the University of Virginia School of Medicine and Elsevier. The University of Virginia School of Medicine is accredited by the ACCME to provide continuing medical education for physicians.

The University of Virginia School of Medicine designates this educational activity for a maximum of 15 *AMA PRA Category 1 Credits*™ for each issue, 60 credits per year. Physicians should only claim credit commensurate with the extent of their participation in the activity.

The American Medical Association has determined that physicians not licensed in the US who participate in this CME activity are eligible for a maximum of 15 *AMA PRA Category 1 Credits*™ for each issue, 60 credits per year.

Credit can be earned by reading the text material, taking the CME examination online at http://www.theclinics.com/home/cme, and completing the evaluation. After taking the test, you will be required to review any and all incorrect answers. Following completion of the test and evaluation, your credit will be awarded and you may print your certificate.

FACULTY DISCLOSURE/CONFLICT OF INTEREST

The University of Virginia School of Medicine, as an ACCME accredited provider, endorses and strives to comply with the Accreditation Council for Continuing Medical Education (ACCME) Standards of Commercial Support, Commonwealth of Virginia statutes, University of Virginia policies and procedures, and associated federal and private regulations and guidelines on the need for disclosure and monitoring of proprietary and financial interests that may affect the scientific integrity and balance of content delivered in continuing medical education activities under our auspices.

The University of Virginia School of Medicine requires that all CME activities accredited through this institution be developed independently and be scientifically rigorous, balanced and objective in the presentation/discussion of its content, theories and practices.

All authors/editors participating in an accredited CME activity are expected to disclose to the readers relevant financial relationships with commercial entities occurring within the past 12 months (such as grants or research support, employee, consultant, stock holder, member of speakers bureau, etc.). The University of Virginia School of Medicine will employ appropriate mechanisms to resolve potential conflicts of interest to maintain the standards of fair and balanced education to the reader. Questions about specific strategies can be directed to the Office of Continuing Medical Education, University of Virginia School of Medicine, Charlottesville, Virginia.

The faculty and staff of the University of Virginia Office of Continuing Medical Education have no financial affiliations to disclose.

The authors/editors listed below have identified no professional or financial affiliations for themselves or their spouse/partner:
Matthew J. Bassignani, MD (Test Author); Richard D. Bellah, MD; Thomas P. Boulden, MD; Michel Claudon, MD; Harris L. Cohen, MD, FACR; Brian D. Coley, MD (Guest Editor); Kassa Darge, MD, PhD; Vikram S. Dogra, MD (Consulting Editor); Barton Dudlick (Acquisitions Editor); Dana Dumitriu, MD; Monica S. Epelman, MD; Marie-Agnès Galloy, MD; Laurent Garel, MD; Elton B. Greene, MD; Jeanne G. Hill, MD; Kathleen M. McCarten, MD, FACR; Marthe M. Munden, MD; and Laura Varich, MD.

The authors/editors listed below have identified the following professional or financial affiliations for themselves or their spouse/partner:
Boaz Karmazyn, MD is an industry funded research/investigator for Simens.

Disclosure of Discussion of Non-FDA Approved Uses for Pharmaceutical Products and/or Medical Devices.
The University of Virginia School of Medicine, as an ACCME provider, requires that all faculty presenters identify and disclose any off-label uses for pharmaceutical and medical device products. The University of Virginia School of Medicine recommends that each physician fully review all the available data on new products or procedures prior to clinical use.

TO ENROLL

To enroll in the Ultrasound Clinics Continuing Medical Education program, call customer service at 1-800-654-2452 or visit us online at www.theclinics.com/home/cme. The CME program is available to subscribers for an additional fee of $205.00.

Preface

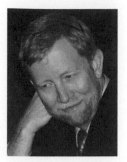

Brian D. Coley, MD
Guest Editor

I hope you enjoyed the October 2009 and January 2010 issues of *Ultrasound Clinics*, which featured articles on pediatric musculoskeletal and head-and-neck applications. This issue focuses on the genitourinary tract and abdomen. It also includes an excellent concluding article about emerging advances and techniques that promise to make ultrasound an even more valuable diagnostic tool for both children and adults. As before, all of the authors are experienced sonologists and have provided excellent material useful for enhancing and expanding your ultrasound practice. Since writing the previous issue's preface, there has been a new wave of concern over medical radiation exposure, this time focusing more on adults. While this attention has produced a certain amount of news hype and hysteria that is sure to wane, the concerns have validity and will provide, I hope, some impetus to radiologists to rediscover the value of ultrasound.

As always, thanks to the great staff at Elsevier and to the publisher of *Ultrasound Clinics*, Barton Dudlick. They have taken care to present the work of the authors in the best manner possible. To the authors of this issue and the previous one, many thanks for taking the time and effort to write, and for writing so well.

Brian D. Coley, MD
Department of Radiology
Nationwide Children's Hospital
700 Children's Drive
Columbus, OH 43205, USA
The Ohio State University
College of Medicine
and Public Health
Columbus, OH, USA

E-mail address:
brian.coley@nationwidechildrens.org

Ultrasound Clin 5 (2010) ix
doi:10.1016/j.cult.2010.01.001

Sonography in the Evaluation of Pediatric Urinary Tract Infection

Richard D. Bellah, MD[a,b,*], Monica S. Epelman, MD[a],
Kassa Darge, MD, PhD[a,c]

KEYWORDS

• Urinary • Infection • Evaluation • Tract • Sonography

Urinary tract infection (UTI) is a common pediatric malady, and a frequent source of morbidity in the pediatric population. The gold standard for the diagnosis of UTI is growth of pathogenic bacteria (commonly *Escherichia coli*, *Klebsiella*, *Proteus*, and *Pseudomonas*) in urine culture. In the outpatient setting, however, rapid techniques (ie, urine dipstick for leukocyte esterase or nitrites) are often used.[1]

Many complex factors play a role in the pathogenesis of UTI in children. When bacterial virulence factors, such as adherence and motility factors, outweigh host resistance factors, UTI is favored to occur.[2,3] Host anatomic, humoral, and genetic factors also play a role. UTIs are highest for both boys and girls during the first year of life, and decrease after that. During the first few months of life, the incidence of UTI in boys exceeds that in girls, likely because of colonization of the prepuce in uncircumcised boys by uropathogenic bacteria.[4] Beyond that, first time and recurrent UTIs are more common in girls. Estimates of rates of infection in the first 24 months of life indicate 3% in boys less than 1 year; 2% in boys greater than 1 year (< 0.5% for circumcised boys); 7% for girls less than 1 year; and 8% for girls 1 to 2 years of age.[5] Some studies have also suggested a greater tendency of UTI in white versus black girls.[6]

The symptoms of UTI in children can be quite varied, depending on whether the infection is confined to the urethra, bladder, or upper urinary tract (ureter, collecting system, or renal parenchyma). The true incidence is unknown, however, because of the nonspecificity or absence of symptoms.[7,8] In the absence of imaging studies, from a clinical standpoint, the febrile infant or child with clinically significant bacteremia and no other sites of infection is assumed to have upper UTI (pyelonephritis). When a child has a UTI and voiding symptoms, little to no fever, and no systemic symptoms, lower UTI (cystitis) is suspected. The distinction is not always clear, however, in young children. The morbidity associated with UTI can be quite varied as a result, ranging from systemic symptoms associated with acute pyelonephritis (APN) to voiding symptoms of cystitis. Although long-term follow-up data are limited, several studies have noted an association between children with renal scarring caused by APN with

[a] Department of Radiology and Pediatrics, University of Pennsylvania School of Medicine, The Children's Hospital of Philadelphia, 34th and Spruce Street, Philadelphia, PA 19104, USA
[b] Division of Ultrasound, The Children's Hospital of Philadelphia, 34th Street and Civic Center Boulevard, Philadelphia, PA 19104, USA
[c] Division of Body Imaging, The Children's Hospital of Philadelphia, 34th Street and Civic Center Boulevard, Philadelphia, PA 19104, USA
* Corresponding author. Department of Radiology and Pediatrics, University of Pennsylvania School of Medicine, The Children's Hospital of Philadelphia, 34th and Spruce Street, Philadelphia, PA 19104.
E-mail address: bellah@email.chop.edu

Ultrasound Clin 5 (2010) 1–13
doi:10.1016/j.cult.2009.11.014
1556-858X/10/$ – see front matter © 2010 Elsevier Inc. All rights reserved.

hypertension and end-stage renal disease.[9,10] Although more recent studies question this association, the high prevalence of and frequent morbidity associated with pediatric UTIs have perpetuated the need for continued examination of the role of imaging in its diagnosis and management.

IMAGING GOALS AND CONSIDERATIONS

The purpose of investigating the child's urinary tract after infection is (1) to discover a possible cause for the infection to prevent recurrence and lessen morbidity; (2) to determine whether the kidneys are normal, involved, or at risk for scarring; (3) to determine whether vesicoureteral reflux (VUR) exists, which facilitates the ascent of infection from the bladder; (4) to identify urinary tract calculi, which may perpetuate or result from repeated UTI; and (5) to identify urine outflow obstruction.[7,8] Although VUR has been considered a major risk factor for UTI and renal damage, it has been shown that UTI and renal scarring can occur without VUR, and that some children with UTI and VUR may never have renal scarring. Imaging strategies, which typically include ultrasound (US), nuclear cortical imaging (with dimercaptosuccinic acid [DMSA]), and voiding cystourethrography (VCUG), are gradually changing. Despite this, many organizations, such as the American College of Radiology and European Society for Pediatric Radiology, to standardize diagnostic imaging tests have offered recommendations and guidelines for evaluating the child with UTI.[11,12] It is recognized, however, that no single imaging technique can address all of the essential questions. Even more confounding, some investigators have recently questioned the use of US in particular, despite its attraction as a noninvasive technique.[13] This is mainly because of its inability to detect inflammatory change, small scarred areas within the kidneys, or intermittent dilatation related to VUR.[14] In one of these studies, which questioned the need for routine US, the sensitivity, specifically, positive predictive value, and negative predictive value of renal US for detecting VUR were 17%, 88%, 24%, and 83%, respectively.[15] In another study, the sensitivity was 10%, and in none of those patients with abnormal renal US was there a need for change in patient management.[16] Nevertheless, because the technical quality of gray-scale and color Doppler US have continued to improve, and newer US techniques are continually developing, radiology organizations and pediatric uroradiology societies continue to include US as an important step in their imaging protocol.[12] Pediatric practitioners remain reluctant to abandon the tradition of routine US because it poses no risk or discomfort to the young patient.[17] The following subsections describe the key basic features of US in the setting of pediatric UTI, and describe the advantages of potential additional US techniques and applications, such as high-resolution US, harmonic imaging, and contrast-enhanced voiding urosonography (VUS).

UTI: US TECHNIQUE AND FINDINGS

US evaluation of the urinary tract in the pediatric patient with UTI should include evaluation of the kidneys; ureters (if visible); and urinary bladder. The highest frequency transducer that penetrates the area should be used. For infants and toddlers, a curved 8- to 13-MHz transducer, for young children, a curved array 4- to 9-MHz transducer, and for adolescents, a 2- to 5-MHz curved array transducer can be used.

For infants and young children, one should first examine the bladder because the infant may empty his or her bladder, rendering it difficult to obtain useful information about the bladder itself; the bladder wall; and distal ureters (their caliber and insertion sites). The bladder should be reasonably well-distended, and examined in transverse and sagittal planes. In the transverse plane, images should be obtained from the bladder dome to the bladder outlet. In the sagittal plane, images should include the bladder outlet, the bilateral distal ureters, and ureteral insertion sites. Color Doppler US can be useful in identifying the latter when ureteral jets are seen.

In the child with UTI, the goal of sonography of the bladder is to provide information that may help to determine why the child may have been predisposed to infection. The bladder wall thickness is usually regarded as normal up to 0.3 cm with a full bladder and 0.5 cm with an empty bladder.[18] Conditions that may cause bladder wall thickening that could predispose the child to infection include bladder outlet obstruction and dysfunctional voiding (with or without neurogenic bladder dysfunction) (Fig. 1). In the child with so-called "dysfunctional elimination syndrome," in addition to voiding dysfunction, constipation may also play a role in the development of UTI.[19] Large bladder diverticula can also result in dysfunctional voiding because of one's inability to completely or effectively empty his or her bladder (Fig. 2). In the acute setting, bladder wall thickening may be caused by cystitis, which may be of bacterial or viral origin. The gray-scale images show irregular bladder wall thickening; color flow Doppler US shows hyperemia of the bladder wall (Fig. 3).[20] Bladder wall thickening in cystitis caused by

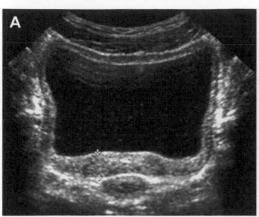
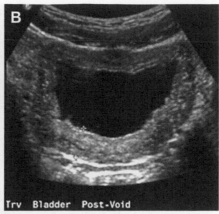

Fig. 1. Dysfunctional elimination syndrome. US of the urinary bladder (transverse) prevoid (A) and postvoid (B) in a 6-year-old girl with frequency, dribbling, and recurrent UTIs shows bladder wall thickening and moderate post-void residual.

adenovirus can be so mass-like in some cases as to mimic bladder tumors (Fig. 4).[21] In addition to determination of bladder functional disturbances, US of the bladder is required for identifying potentially associated urinary tract abnormalities, such as ureteral ectopy, ureteroceles, or megaureter. In so doing, the distal ureters are assessed for caliber and insertion sites. Low-level echoes or internal debris within a dilated lumen can indicate superimposed infection or pyoureteronephrosis (Fig. 5).[22]

Conventional gray-scale US of the distal ureters and the pelvicalyceal system is generally regarded as a poor screening method for the detection of VUR.[23] Hoberman and colleagues[16] studied 309 children, aged 1 to 24 months, using US, DMSA, and VCUG, and found the sensitivity of US for detecting VUR on VCUG was 10% and positive predictive value was 40%. VUR detection may be improved with meticulous or advanced US techniques. Contrast-enhanced VUS, which uses intravesical US contrast agent, is gaining widespread application, particularly in Europe, as a radiation-free alternative to the conventional radiologic VUR diagnostic modalities, VCUG, and radionuclide cystography.[24] Taking VCUG as the reference standard, studies of VUS for VUR detection have shown the following: sensitivity 57% to 100%, specificity 85% to 100%, positive and negative predictive values 58% to 100% and 87% to 100%, and diagnostic accuracy 78% to 96%. Attempts are underway to introduce VUS in Canada, where the appropriate contrast agents are already available.[25] In the United States, however, lack of suitable Food and Drug Administration–approved US contrast agents for children have held back its introduction. VUS encompasses the following four basic steps[26–28]: (1) precontrast examination, standard US of the urinary tract in supine (± prone) position; (2) catheterization or suprapubic puncture of the bladder under sterile condition and administration of normal saline and US contrast agent; (3) postcontrast examination, a repeat of the standard US of the urinary tract; and (4) postcontrast voiding examination, US of the renal pelves and terminal ureters (± urethra) during and after voiding. Reflux is diagnosed when echogenic microbubbles are detected in the ureters or pelvicalyceal system. During the postcontrast examinations the right and left renal pelves are scanned alternatively. The scan during voiding can be performed when the patient is lying, sitting on a bedpan, or standing and voiding into a urine bottle. The severity of reflux is graded in a similar manner as the international reflux grading system for VCUG (grades 1–5).[26]

Depending on the availability, different US imaging modalities are used in VUS to depict the refluxing microbubbles. The imaging options not only affect the conspicuity of the microbubbles but also the overall diagnostic accuracy of the examination. Conventional (fundamental) US has been widely used for VUS. It can be combined with color Doppler to enhance the detection of reflux. When using harmonic imaging, microbubbles become strikingly more conspicuous compared with fundamental mode, with increased sensitivity for reflux detection.[29] The most advanced modalities of choice for VUS, which have brought about a profound improvement in detecting refluxing microbubbles, use advanced contrast-specific imaging modalities tuned for individual contrast agents using low or high mechanical index.

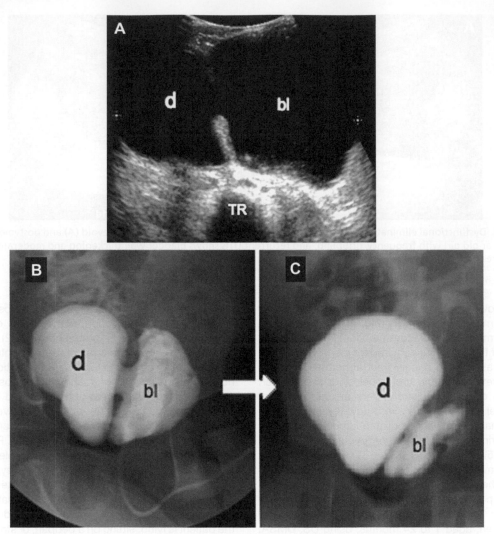

Fig. 2. Large bladder diverticulum resulting in incomplete bladder emptying. (*A*) US (trans) of the bladder (bl) demonstrates a large right-sided bladder diverticulum (d). (*B, C*) VCUG shows a large right bladder diverticulum (d), which increases in size during voiding, resulting in incomplete bladder emptying.

The microbubbles are not only enhanced and color-coded, but it is also possible to visualize only the refluxing microbubbles blocking out the background gray-scale image (**Fig. 6**). Compared with VCUG, the potential drawbacks of VUS are (1) urethral sonography is performed in just a few centers and has not yet found widespread acceptance, (2) longer examination duration, and (3) limitation of bladder function evaluation.[29]

US of the kidneys has several purposes in the initial evaluation of the child with UTI, mainly to detect structural abnormalities (congenital or acquired). In the acute setting, in which an infant or child is diagnosed with UTI, the purpose of the renal US examination is to determine if the kidneys are infected, and to detect preexisting abnormalities of the kidneys that could predispose them to infection. These may include obstructive uropathies; urolithiasis; anomalies of renal size; position or shape; and duplication of a collecting system with ureteral ectopy, with or without ureterocele. Renal length (and volumes) should be obtained routinely and compared with normal values according to patient age, weight, and possibly body surface area.[30] The prone sagittal views of the kidneys are the most readily reproducible planes for measurements of renal length, because renal length can vary on US according to patient position.[31] Renal enlargement in APN can be quite variable. Initially, the renal volume may be normal but later increases as the inflammatory process progresses.[32] Renal enlargement

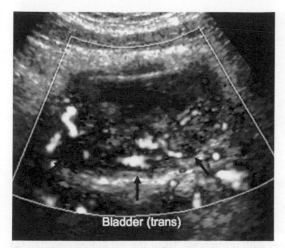

Fig. 3. Bacterial cystitis. Color flow Doppler US of the bladder (transverse) shows severe irregular bladder wall thickening with hyperemia of the bladder base (*arrows*).

can be focal or global, in the latter instance ranging from 120% to 175% of normal size (**Fig. 7**).[33] Renal enlargement may not be apparent on US 1 to 2 weeks after presentation once the infection has cleared.[11] In addition to unilateral or bilateral renal enlargement, other findings that can be seen, particularly in severe infections, include loss of corticomedullary differentiation, and localized areas of hypoechogenic or hyperechogenic renal parenchyma (**Fig. 8**). Thickening of the uroepithelium of the renal pelvicalyceal system or ureters may be seen in infection (pyelitis) and with VUR (see **Fig. 7**).[34] Harmonic imaging accentuates posterior shadowing, acoustic enhancement, or comet tail artifacts, and can also provide improved image quality and resolution of small renal lesions (**Fig. 9**).[35] Contrast resolution and lateral resolution can also be improved with harmonic imaging, and in pediatric urologic imaging harmonic imaging is particularly superior to conventional US when

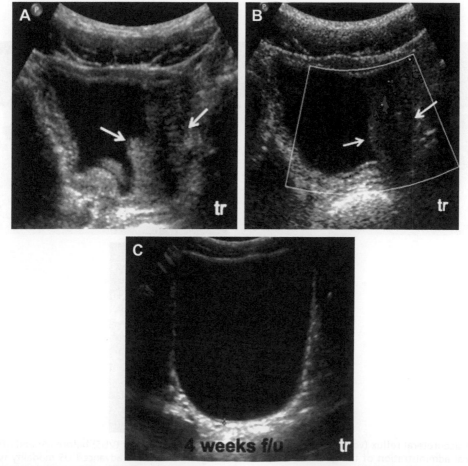

Fig. 4. Viral cystitis mimicking bladder mass. Gray-scale (*A*) and color flow Doppler (*B*) US of the bladder demonstrates an irregular mass-like thickening with hyperemia involving the left aspect of the bladder wall (*arrows*). (*C*) US of the bladder at 4-week follow-up shows resolution of focal bladder wall thickening.

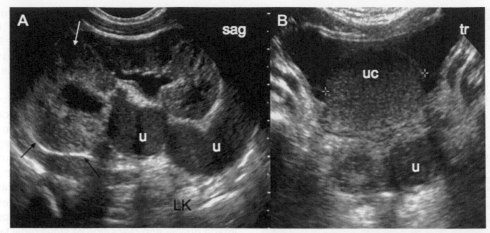

Fig. 5. Pyoureteronephrosis (upper pole) in a duplex kidney with ureterocele. US of the left kidney (sagittal) (A) and bladder (transverse) (B) show dilated echogenic upper pole moiety (arrows), dilated ureter (u), and ureterocele (uc) containing internal echoes.

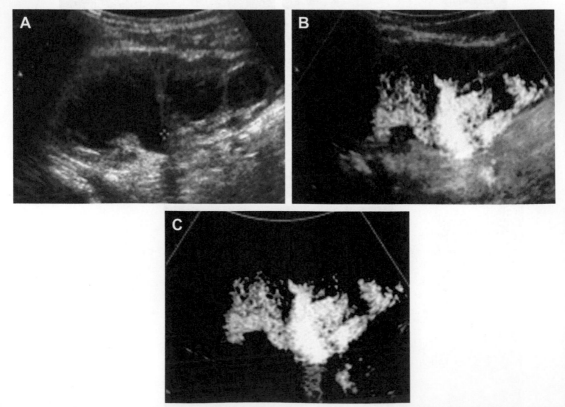

Fig. 6. Vesicoureteral reflux (voiding urosonography). Voiding urosonography (VUS) before (A) and after (B, C) intravesical administration of the galactose-based contrast agent. Dedicated advanced US modality with high mechanical index is used for the study. (A) The kidney demonstrates marked pelvicalyceal dilatation and cortical thinning. The refluxing microbubbles are depicted with color overlay and without (B) and with subtraction of the gray-scale background (C).

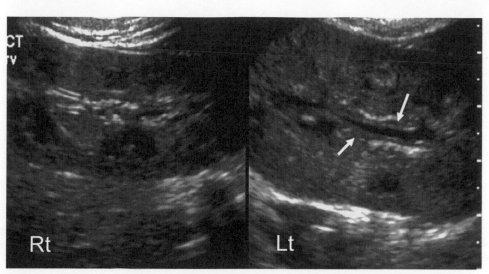

Fig. 7. Acute pyelonephritis, diffuse. US of the bilateral kidneys demonstrate a normal right kidney. The left kidney is globally enlarged and increased in its overall echogenicity. There is loss of normal corticomedullary differentiation. Note thickening of the uroepithelium of the renal pelvis (*arrows*).

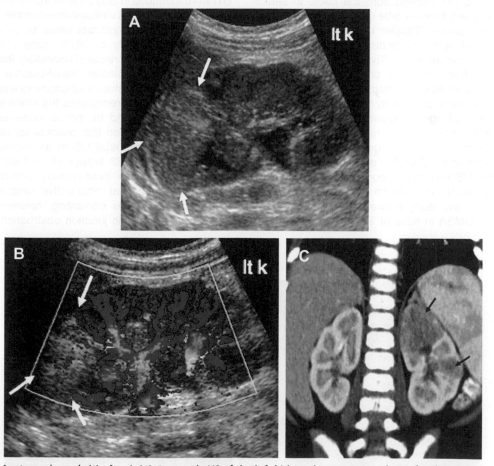

Fig. 8. Acute pyelonephritis, focal. (*A*) Gray-scale US of the left kidney demonstrates a large focal area (*arrows*) of hyperechogenicity and loss of corticomedullary differentiation in the upper pole of the left kidney. (*B*) Color flow Doppler image demonstrates marked decreased flow within the affected echogenic upper pole (*arrows*). (*C*) Contrast CT (coronal reconstruction) confirms focal APN in left upper pole and smaller area in midpole (*arrows*) of left kidney.

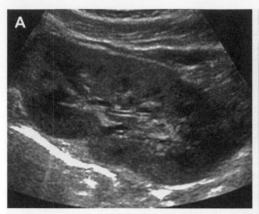
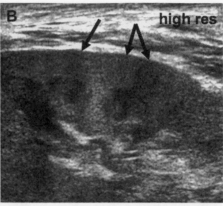

Fig. 9. Acute pyelonephritis, high-resolution US. (*A*) US (sagittal) of the left kidney with curvilinear array trans-ducer shows normal cortical echogenicity, corticomedullary differentiation, and no focal abnormalities. (*B*) Linear high-resolution image shows multifocal regions (*arrows*) of striated cortical hypoechogenicity, compatible with APN.

examining the kidneys from the back. In select cases, when there is little (patient) motion, color flow and power Doppler US may improve the ability to detect APN by displaying areas of poor or absent perfusion.[36,37] These areas of hypoper-fusion reflect vasculitis or vasoconstriction of peripheral arterioles related to bacterial infection (**Fig. 10**). This is particularly helpful in infants under 3 months of age, in whom the use of Tc-99m DMSA scintigraphy, the reference standard for the evaluation of APN, is generally discouraged.[6] In general, in the detection of APN without compli-cations, US compares poorly with imaging stan-dards, such as Tc-99m DMSA scintigraphy (**Fig. 11**). One study showed that abnormal find-ings by DMSA in 63% of 91 children with acute

UTI were identified in only 24% of the same group by US.[38] Because it is well documented that febrile UTIs in children may indicate either an underlying anatomic abnormality or VUR, many clinicians believe that renal US remains necessary following a first febrile UTI episode. Renal-bladder US is most often the initial study that uncovers an under-lying condition that predisposes the infant or child to infection. It should be noted, however, that some authors question this practice for patients who underwent prenatal US in an experienced center after 30 to 32 weeks of gestation.[17] In most instances, the predisposing condition is a form of congenital obstructive uropathy or high-grade VUR. It is interesting, however, that although ureteropelvic junction obstruction is the

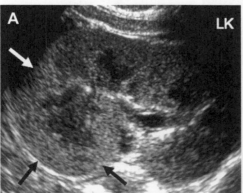
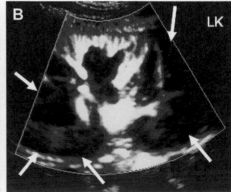

Fig. 10. Acute pyelonephritis, power Doppler US. (*A*) Gray-scale US demonstrates subtle increase in the echoge-nicity of the upper pole of the left kidney (*arrows*). (*B*) Power Doppler US demonstrates diminished perfusion in the upper and lower poles (*arrows*) of the left kidney compatible with multifocal APN.

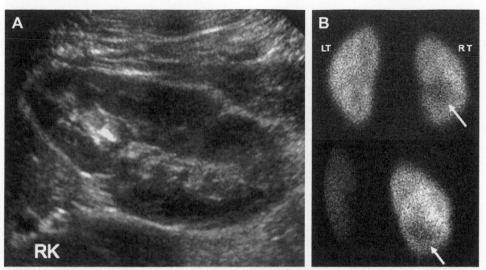

Fig. 11. Acute pyelonephritis, US/DMSA. (*A*) US of the right kidney shows normal cortical echogenicity, cortico-medullary differentiation, and no focal abnormalities. (*B*) Contemporaneous DMSA (posterior view) shows photopenic area in the mid-lower pole of the left kidney (*arrows*) compatible with APN.

most common form of congenital urinary tract obstruction, from personal observation ureteropelvic junction obstruction is rarely noted to be the underlying condition responsible for the development of UTI in children. Pyoureteronephrosis, in which infection or purulent material appears as low-level echoes within the dilated collecting systems, seems to favor such conditions as megaureter and duplex kidneys with either ureteral ectopy or ureterocele, which are associated with ureteral dilatation (see **Fig. 5**). Under certain circumstances, such as prematurity or usage of long-term antibiotics, renal fungal infection may occur and appear as casts or clumps of echogenic material (fungal balls) within dilated upper collecting systems (**Fig. 12**).[39] In rare instances, *E coli* toxin can produce ureteral atony resulting in ureteral dilatation alone.

US may detect complications related to APN, such as renal abscess, perinephric abscess, xanthogranulomatous pyelonephritis, and renal stones (**Fig. 13**). Abscesses may be single or multiple, and result from APN or hematogenous infection. Small parenchymal or perinephric abscesses may be difficult to visualize at grayscale US; larger abscesses appear as well-circumscribed hypoechoic collections with internal echoes. In most of these instances, the US examination can be complemented by additional cross-sectional imaging modalities that may be useful in guidance for intervention (**Fig. 14**). Perinephric abscesses typically result from rupture of cortical

abscesses into the adjacent perinephric soft tissues.

Another role of the initial renal US examination, not necessarily in the acute setting, is to determine whether the kidneys demonstrate acquired abnormalities, such as parenchymal scarring, caused by prior unsuspected or unrecognized kidney infections. Significant focal cortical thinning may be suggested if the renal sinus echoes (fat) reaches the cortical margins of the affected kidney; this finding is most often apparent at the renal poles

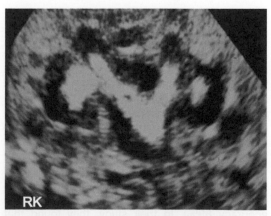

Fig. 12. Renal candidiasis (neonate). US (coronal) of the right kidney in a premature infant demonstrates a cast of echogenic material within the mildly dilated intrarenal pelvicalyceal system.

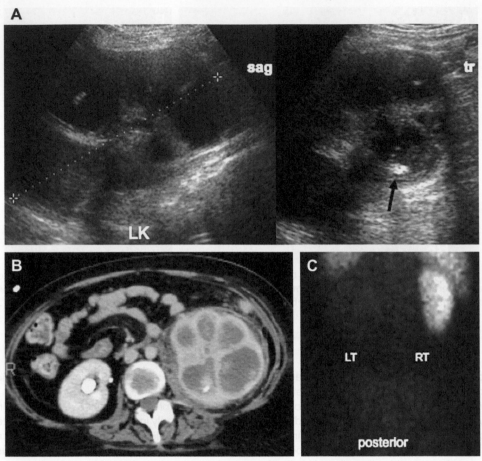

Fig. 13. Xanthogranulomatous pyelonephritis. (*A*) US of the left kidney (sagittal, transverse) demonstrates left renal enlargement with large hypoechoic regions secondary to moderately severe caliectasis. A small calculus (*arrow*) is seen within the left renal pelvis. (*B*) Delayed-contrast CT shows a normal right kidney, left renal enlargement with inflammatory changes in Gerota fascia, minimal cortical enhancement without excretion, severe caliectasis, and a small renal calculus. (*C*) Tc-99m Mag-3 renal scintigraphy (posterior view) demonstrates nonfunctioning left kidney and normal functioning right kidney.

(Fig. 15). Small- and medium-sized scars are not as readily detected with US. The degree of cortical thinning may be severe enough to result in renal size disparity. As with APN, DMSA is regarded as the goal standard for the detection of renal scarring.[40,41] Only approximately 4% of children have visible parenchymal defects as a result of UTI that are visible by DMSA scan.[42] In a study by Luk and coworkers[42] of 55 children with renal scarring by DMSA, 29% had abnormal US findings (sensitivity 29%, positive predictive value 41%, accuracy 89%). In their study, they found that the negative predictive value of US, combined with VCUG, was high in predicting absence of scarring, and suggest that DMSA is not necessary

in children less than 2 years of age, if the US and VCUG are normal. Similarly, Christian and colleagues[43] examined the risk of missing renal cortical scarring, detectable on DMSA scintigraphy, if US alone is used, factoring for clinical features (upper or lower tract), UTI recurrence, and age group. They found the risks of missing scarring, detectable on DMSA, varied between 0.4% (in school-age children with solitary lower tract UTI) and 11% (in infants with recurrent upper tract UTI). As with US, however, the role of DMSA scintigraphy is also evolving.[17] Placing the emphasis on renal scarring, some authors suggest that children less than 2 years age with well-documented UTI should have US to exclude underlying

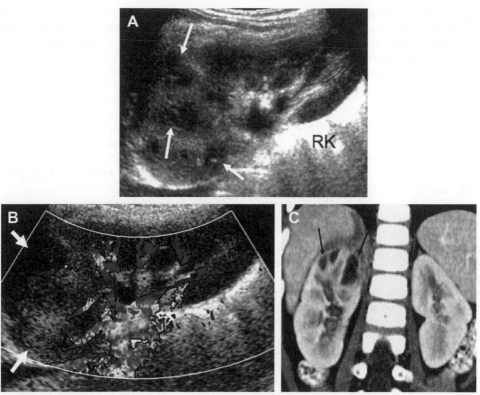

Fig. 14. Acute pyelonephritis with renal abscesses. (*A*) US (sagittal) of the right kidney shows right renal enlargement, with loss of normal upper pole architecture with multiple focal hypoechoic areas (*arrows*). (*B*) Color Doppler US shows marked decreased perfusion of the upper pole (*arrows*). (*C*) Contrast CT (coronal recon) shows APN with multifocal abscesses (*arrows*) in the right upper pole.

anatomic problems and DMSA scintigraphy to exclude renal scarring and possibly the need for VCUG.[7,44,45]

SUMMARY

In the past decade, the imaging approach to pediatric UTI has been challenged by evidence-based literature and physician experience. Among the practice guidelines being questioned that involve each of the imaging modalities, the routine use of US for first-time uncomplicated pediatric UTI evaluation has become controversial.[17] This is the result of several studies having shown that US provides low yield for additional clinically useful information.[13–16] Nevertheless, for all of its

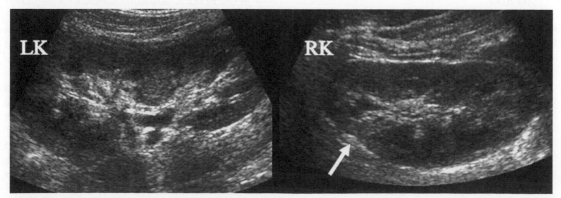

Fig. 15. Chronic pyelonephritis. US of the bilateral kidneys demonstrates a focal area of cortical thinning (*arrow*) within the upper pole of the right kidney (the left kidney is normal).

advantages, including its use for depicting structural urinary tract abnormalities, many pediatric practioners have continued to include US as an integral part of their routine evaluation of first-time UTI in pediatric patients.[1,12,17]

REFERENCES

1. Zorc JJ, Kiddoo DA, Shaw KN. Diagnosis and management of pediatric urinary tract infections. Clin Microbiol Rev 2005;18(2):417–22.
2. Svanborg-Eden C, Hagberg L, Hull R, et al. Bacterial virulence versus host resistance in the urinary tracts of mice. Infect Immun 1987;55:1224–32.
3. Roberts JA. Factors predisposing to urinary tract infections in children. Pediatr Nephrol 1996;10: 517–22.
4. Wiswell TE, Miller GM, Gelston HM, et al. Effect of circumcision status on periurethral bacterial flora during the first year of life. J Pediatr 1988;113(3): 442–6.
5. Downs SM. Technical report: urinary tract infections in febrile infants and young children. The Urinary Tract Subcommittee of the American Academy of Pediatrics Committee on Quality Improvement. Pediatrics 1999;103(4):e54.
6. Shaw K, Gorelick K, McGowan N, et al. Prevalence of urinary tract infection in febrile young children in the emergency department. Pediatrics 1998;102: e16.
7. Smith EA. Pyelonephritis, renal scarring, and reflux nephropathy: a pediatric urologist's perspective. Pediatr Radiol 2008;38(Suppl 1):S76–82.
8. Paltiel HJ. Ultrasound: a practical approach to clinical problems. In: Bluth E, editor. New York: Thieme; 2008. p. 500–13.
9. Jacobsen SH, Eklof AC, Eriksson CG, et al. Development of hypertension and uremia after pyelonephritis in childhood: 27 year follow up. BMJ 1989; 299:703–6.
10. Smellie JM, Prescd NP, Shaw PJ, et al. Childhood reflux and urinary tract infection: a follow-up of 10-41 years in 226 adults. Pediatr Nephrol 1998;12: 727–36.
11. Podbersky DJ, Unsell BJ, Gunderman R, et al. Expert panel on pediatric imaging: urinary tract infection—child [online publication]. Reston (VA): American College of Radiology (ACR); 2006. p. 7.
12. Riccabona M, Avni FE, Blickman JG, et al. Imaging recommendations in paediatric uroradiology: minutes of the ESPR workgroup session on urinary tract infection, fetal hydronephrosis, urinary tract ultrasonography, and voiding cystourethrography, Barcelona Spain, 2007. Pediatr Radiol 2008;38: 138–45.
13. Alon US, Ganapathy S. Should renal ultrasonography be done routinely in children with first urinary tract infection? Clin Pediatr (Phila) 1999;38:21–5.
14. Smellie JM, Rigden SPA, Prescod NP. Urinary tract infection: a comparison of four methods of investigation. Arch Dis Child 1995;72(3):247–50.
15. Zamir G, Sakran W, Horowitz Y, et al. Urinary tract infection: is there a need for routine renal ultrasonography? Arch Dis Child 2004;89:466–8.
16. Hoberman A, Charron M, Hickey RW, et al. Imaging studies after a first febrile urinary tract infection in young children. N Engl J Med 2003; 348(3):195–202.
17. Lim R. Vesicoureteral reflux and urinary tract infection: evolving practices and current controversies in pediatric imaging. AJR Am J Roentgenol 2009; 192:1197–208.
18. Jequier S, Rousseau O. Sonographic measurements of the normal bladder wall in children. AJR Am J Roentgenol 1987;149:563–6.
19. O'Regan S, Yazbeck S, Schick E. Constipation, bladder instability, urinary tract infection syndrome. Clin Nephrol 1985;23:152–4.
20. Gooding GA. Varied sonographic manifestations of cystitis. J Ultrasound Med 1986;5:61–3.
21. Friedman EP, de Bruyn R, Mather S. Pseudotumoral cystitis in children: a review of the ultrasound features in four cases. Br J Radiol 1993;66(787): 605–8.
22. Jeffrey RB Jr, Laing FC, Wing VW, et al. Sensitivity of sonography in pyonephrosis: a reevaluation. AJR Am J Roentgenol 1985;144:71–3.
23. Evans D, Meyer J, Harty P, et al. Assessment of increase in renal pelvic size on post-void sonography as a predictor of vesicoureteral reflux. Pediatr Radiol 1999;29(4):291–4.
24. Darge K, Zieger B, Rohrschneider W, et al. Reduction in voiding cystourethrographies after the introduction of contrast enhanced sonographic reflux diagnosis. Pediatr Radiol 2001;31:790–5.
25. Schneider K, Helmig FJ, Eife R, et al. Pyonephrosis in childhood: is ultrasound sufficient for diagnosis? Pediatr Radiol 1989;19(5):302–7.
26. Berrocal T, Gaya F, Arjonilla A, et al. Vesicoureteral reflux: diagnosis and grading with echo-enhanced cystosonography versus voiding cystourethrography. Radiology 2001;221:359–65.
27. Darge K. Voiding urosonography with ultrasound contrast agents for the diagnosis of vesicoureteric reflux in children. I Procedure. Pediatr Radiol 2008; 38:40–53.
28. Darge K. Voiding urosonography with ultrasound contrast agents for the diagnosis of vesicoureteric reflux in children. II Procedure. Pediatr Radiol 2008;38:54–63.
29. Darge K, Moeller RT, Trusen A, et al. Diagnosis of vesicoureteral reflux with low-dose contrast

enhanced harmonic ultrasound imaging. Pediatr Radiol 2004;35:73–8.

30. Han BK, Babcock DS. Sonographic measurements and appearance of normal kidneys in children. AJR Am J Roentgenol 1985;145:611–6.

31. Carrici CW, Zerin JM. Sonographic measurement of renal length in children: does the position of the patient matter? Pediatr Radiol 1996;26:553–5.

32. Sty JR, Wells RG, Starshak RJ, et al. Imaging in acute renal infection in children. AJR Am J Roentgenol 1987;148:471–7.

33. Dinkel E, Orth S, Dittrich M, et al. Renal sonography in the differentiation of upper from lower urinary tract infection. AJR Am J Roentgenol 1986;146(4):775–80.

34. Avni EF, Van Gansbeke D, Thoua Y, et al. US demonstration of pyelitis and ureteritis in children. Pediatr Radiol 1988;18:134–9.

35. Bartram U, Darge K. Harmonic versus conventional ultrasound imaging of the urinary tract in children. Pediatr Radiol 2005;35:655–60.

36. Winters WD. Power Doppler sonographic evaluation of acute pyelonephritis in children. J Ultrasound Med 1996;15(2):91–6.

37. Dacher JN, Pfister C, Monroc M, et al. Power Doppler sonographic pattern of acute pyelonephritis in children: comparison with CT. AJR Am J Roentgenol 1996;166(6):1451–5.

38. Björgvinsson E, Majd M, Eggli KD. Diagnosis of acute pyelonephritis in children: comparison of sonography and ^{99m}Tc-DMSA scintigraphy. AJR Am J Roentgenol 1991;157(3):539–43.

39. Cohen HL, Haller JO, Schechter S, et al. Renal candidiasis of the infant: ultrasound evaluation. Urol Radiol 1986;8:17–21.

40. Majd M, Rushton HG. Renal cortical scintigraphy in the diagnosis of acute pyelonephritis. Semin Nucl Med 1992;22(2):98–111.

41. Rushton HG. The evaluation of acute pyelonephritis and renal scarring with technetium 99m-dimercaptosuccinic acid renal scintigraphy: evolving concepts and future directions. Pediatr Nephrol 1997;11(1): 108–20.

42. Luk WH, Woo YH, San Au-Yeung AW, et al. Imaging in pediatric urinary tract infection: a 9-year local experience. AJR Am J Roentgenol 2009;192:1253–60.

43. Christian MT, McColl JH, MacKenzie JR, et al. Risk assessment of renal cortical scarring with urinary tract infection by clinical features and ultrasonography. Arch Dis Child 2000;82(5):376–80.

44. Rushton HG, Pohl HG. Urinary tract infections in children. In: Belman AB, King LR, Kramer SA, editors. Clinical pediatric urology. 4th edition. London: Martin Dunitz; 2002. p. 261.

45. Pohl HG, Belman AB. The top-down approach to the evaluation of children with febrile urinary tract infection. Adv Urol 2009. [Epub ahead of print].

Renal Cystic Disease

Laurent Garel, MD[a,b,*]

KEYWORDS

- Renal cysts • Children • Ultrasound
- Polycystic kidney diseases • Renal dysplasia
- Prenatal imaging

Renal cystic diseases encompass numerous congenital, developmental, or acquired conditions that share the presence of cysts (epithelium-lined cavities filled with fluid or semisolid matter) in one or both kidneys. Cystic kidneys of different etiologies may appear morphologically similar, whereas a spectrum of abnormalities may be imaged in different patients with the same etiologic entity (eg, as in autosomal-recessive polycystic kidney disease [ARPKD]).

Several classifications of renal cysts have been proposed, taking into account pathologic,[1,2] clinical,[3] and genetic features.[4,5] Classifications are likely to evolve, in relation to the better knowledge of the underlying pathogenesis of cyst formation. Recently, the importance of the cilium of the tubular epithelial cell has been recognized as an essential structure in maintaining epithelial cell differentiation. Accordingly, defects in the primary apical cilia of tubular epithelia may play a key role in cystogenesis.[6–11]

CLASSIFICATION OF RENAL CYSTIC DISEASES

From a practical standpoint, it is clinically appropriate to differentiate hereditary cystic kidney disorders from nongenetic renal cysts (**Box 1**). Such a dual classification is especially valuable for the sonologists who image renal cysts in fetuses, infants, children, and adults.[12–14]

For consistency in this article, every condition is addressed by its prevalence; gene mutation; clinical features; natural history; and sonographic pattern (kidney size; overall echogenicity; preservation or not of corticomedullary differentiation; cysts size, number, location, associated features).

HEREDITARY DISORDERS
Autosomal-Dominant Polycystic Kidney Disease

Prevalence
The prevalence of autosomal-dominant polycystic kidney disease (ADPKD) is estimated to be between 1 in 400 and 1 in 1000 live births.

Genetics
ADPKD is an autosomal-dominant inherited trait with almost 100% penetrance. Parents' ultrasound (US) work-up in fetal and pediatric cases of ADPKD has shown a high spontaneous mutation rate, quoted between 5% and 10% depending on series. The 10% figure correlates better with my own experience.

Two genes have been identified: PKD_1 on chromosome 16p (85% of cases) and PKD_2 on chromosome 4q (15% of cases). A PKD_3 gene is suspected but not yet identified. So far, all fetal cases of ADPKD have been PKD_1.

ADPKD shows large interfamilial and intrafamilial variability. Because of variable expressivity

[a] Department of Radiology, Radio-oncology and Nuclear Medicine, University of Montreal, 2900 Edouard-Montpetit Boulevard, Montreal, QC H3T 1J4, Canada
[b] Department of Medical Imaging, Sainte-Justine Mother and Child University Hospital Center, 3175 Cote Ste-Catherine Road, Montreal, QC H3T 1C5, Canada
* Department of Medical Imaging, Sainte-Justine Mother and Child University Hospital Center, 3175 Cote Ste-Catherine Road, Montreal, QC H3T 1C5, Canada.
E-mail address: laurent_garel@ssss.gouv.qc.ca

Ultrasound Clin 5 (2010) 15–59
doi:10.1016/j.cult.2009.11.018
1556-858X/10/$ – see front matter © 2010 Elsevier Inc. All rights reserved.

Classification of renal cysts

Genetic (hereditary) disorders

■ Polycystic kidney disease (autosomal dominant, autosomal recessive)
■ Medullary cystic disease (eg, nephronophthisis)
■ Glomerulocystic kidney disease (autosomal dominant, sporadic)
■ Malformation syndromes (eg, Meckel-Gruber, Bardet-Biedl, tuberous sclerosis)
■ Microcystic kidney disease (congenital nephrotic syndrome)

Nongenetic conditions

■ Renal cystic dysplasia (multicystic dysplastic kidney, obstructive renal dysplasia)
■ Nongenetic, nondysplastic cysts

  – simple cyst
  – medullary sponge kidney
  – renal cystic neoplasms (eg, multilocular cystic nephroma)
  – "acquired" cysts (eg, chronic renal failure)
  – renal cysts of nontubular origin (eg, renal sinus cyst, pyelocalyceal cysts)

and spontaneous mutation, a family history is lacking in nearly 50% of pediatric patients at presentation.

Pathology

Any segment of the nephrons and collecting ducts may be affected. Initially, most cysts in ADPKD arise from the distal part of the nephron and the collecting duct. In more advanced disease, cysts are scattered within the cortex and the medulla. Although bilateral presentation is the norm, 17% of cases are asynchronous or asymmetric, especially in children.[15] Up to 90% of adults with ADPKD have liver cysts. Very rare in the pediatric age group, the frequency of hepatic cysts increases with age; MR imaging prevalence in the Consortium for Radiologic Imaging Studies of PKD cohort study[16] was 58% in the 15- to 24-year-old group. Cysts can also be seen in the pancreas (5% of patients); the arachnoid (8%); and the seminal vesicles (40%). In my experience, extrarenal cysts in children with ADPKD are exceedingly rare.

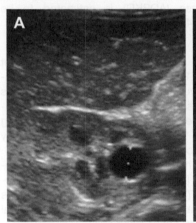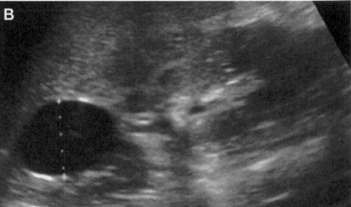

Fig. 1. Three-year-old boy investigated for urinary tract infection. No family history of cystic renal disease. US shows the classical features of ADPKD with bilateral cysts (*cursors*). (*A*) Right kidney (transverse). (*B*) Left kidney (longitudinal).

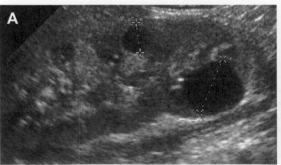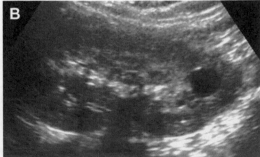

Fig. 2. Mother with known ADPKD. (*A*) Longitudinal sonogram of her child at 4 months of age shows two cysts (*cursors*) within the right kidney. The left kidney was normal. (*B*) At 3 years of age, a newly formed cyst is now visible in the lower pole of the left kidney.

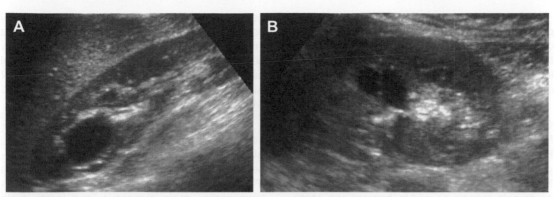

Fig. 3. Eight-year-old girl whose mother and sister have ADPKD. Sonograms of the right kidney (*A*) (longitudinal) and left kidney (*B*) (transverse) show bilateral renal cysts classic for ADPKD.

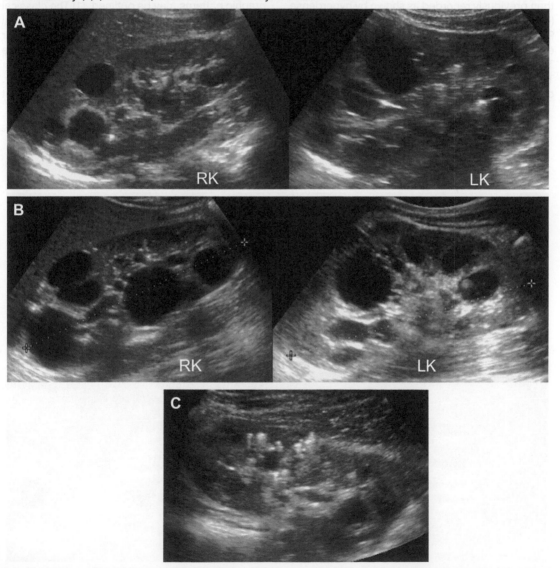

Fig. 4. ADPKD with progression of involvement on two examinations. (*A*) At 9 years of age, the left kidney measures 10 cm, the right kidney 11 cm. Multiple, bilateral cysts are present in the cortex and medulla. (*B*) At 13 years of age, the left kidney measures 13.1 cm, the right kidney 12.7 cm. The cysts have progressed in number and size. (*C*) Comet-tail artifacts most likely represent milk of calcium within the cysts.

Vascular involvement in ADPKD includes intra-cranial aneurysms, thoracic aorta dissection, and coronary artery aneurysms. Widespread presymptomatic screening of intracranial aneurysms is not indicated in the absence of a family history of aneurysm or subarachnoid hemorrhage.

Clinical features and natural history

Most children with ADPKD are asymptomatic.[17,18] Hypertension is present in approximately 50% of young adults (20–34 years old) with ADPKD. Pain is the most common symptom in adult patients; acute pain may be caused by hemorrhage, stone, or infection. Cyst hemorrhage is more frequent than previously recorded as shown by hyperdense (CT) or high-signal (MR imaging) cysts in more than 90% of adult ADPKD patients. Kidney stones are encountered in approximately 20% of adult cases. The development of renal failure is highly variable. The mutated gene (PKD$_1$ vs PKD$_2$), the position of the mutation in PKD$_1$, along with modifiers genes have a significant impact on the clinical course of the disease. Consortium for Radiologic Imaging Studies of PKD has shown that kidney and cyst volumes are the best predictors of renal function impairment.[19–21] Early recognition of ADPKD in fetuses and infants is not correlated with a more severe outcome.[22]

Sonographic features

ADPKD in children presents variably on US, depending mostly on patient age and gene mutation (Figs. 1–17).[14,23,24] Children with PKD$_1$ mutations have earlier, more numerous, and larger cysts than children with PKD$_2$ mutation.[23] Three sonographic patterns may be outlined. (1) The classical form is made of normal-size kidneys with normal parenchymal echogenicity and a limited number of cysts in cortical or medullary location (see Figs. 1–5). US of the parents can be of great interest in the absence of a positive family history. A negative renal sonogram in both parents does not

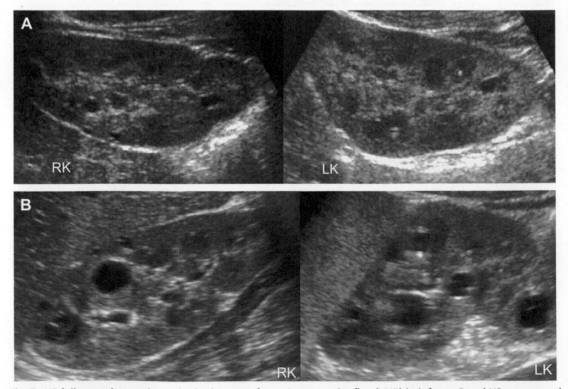

Fig. 5. US follow-up in a patient who had surgery for vesicoureteral reflux (VUR) in infancy. Renal US was normal until the age of 6 years (not shown). US of both parents were normal. There was no significant family history. (*A*) Longitudinal sonograms of both kidneys at 6 years of age show small cysts. (*B*) At 11 years of age, the ADPKD pattern is obvious in both kidneys.

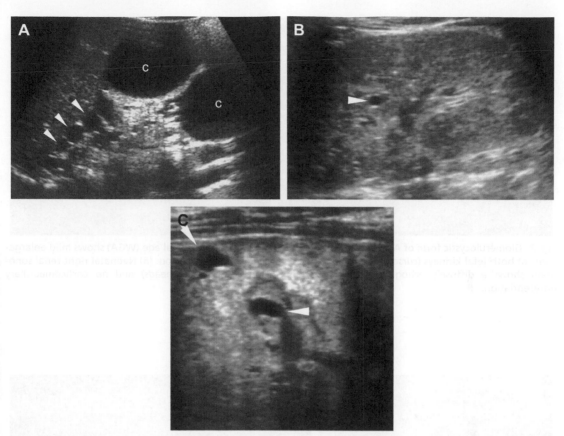

Fig. 6. ADPKD with asymmetric involvement. (*A*) Before 7 years of age, cysts were only visible in the right kidney (two macrocysts in lower pole [C], multiple cysts in upper pole [*arrowheads*]). (*B*) After 7 years of age, evidence of early cystic involvement was noted in the left kidney (*arrowhead*). (*C*) High-resolution US of left kidney at 8 years of age shows a small cyst in the cortex (*arrow*) and in the medulla (*arrowhead*).

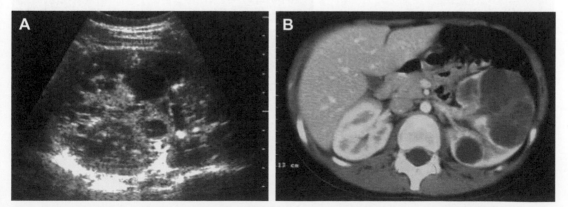

Fig. 7. Unilateral ADPKD in a 10-year-old girl investigated for posttraumatic hematuria. (*A*) US of the left kidney shows multiple cysts and parenchymal distortion. The right kidney was normal. (*B*) Contrast-enhanced CT shows a large cystic mass effect in the left kidney and a normal right kidney. The left kidney was surgically removed and pathology proved the unilateral ADPKD. There was no family history, and US of both parents were normal.

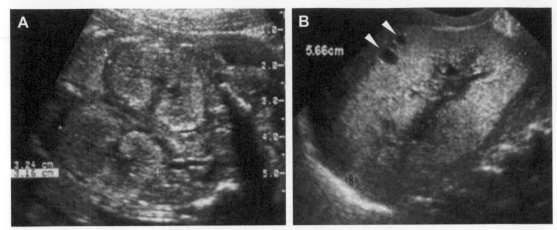

Fig. 8. Glomerulocystic form of ADPKD. (*A*) Obstetric US at 22 weeks gestational age (WGA) shows mild enlargement of both fetal kidneys (*cursors*) with loss of corticomedullary differentiation. (*B*) Neonatal right renal sonogram shows a diffusely echogenic kidney with subcapsular cysts (*arrowheads*) and no corticomedullary differentiation.

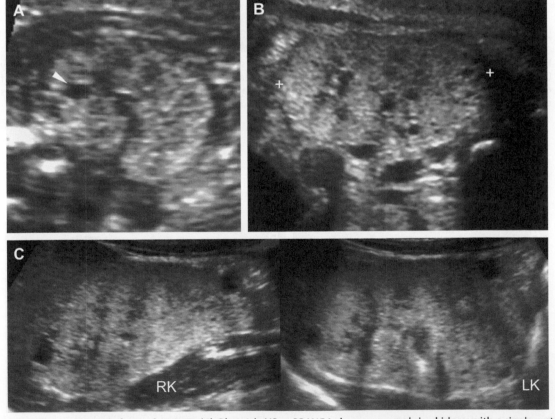

Fig. 9. Glomerulocystic form of ADPKD. (*A*) Obstetric US at 22 WGA shows a normal size kidney with a single cyst (*arrowhead*). (*B*) Obstetric US at 36 WGA shows a moderately enlarged kidney (*cursors*) (60 mm) with absent corticomedullary differentiation and multiple microcysts. (*C*) Renal ultrasound at 5 weeks of age shows mildly enlarged bright kidneys with subcapsular cysts.

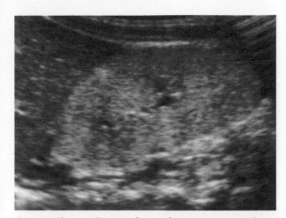

Fig. 10. Glomerulocystic form of ADPKD in a newborn with positive family history (father). Renal US at birth shows a globally hyperechoic kidney without visible subcapsular cysts.

rule out ADPKD because of the 10% fresh mutation rate. Initially, the renal involvement is asymmetric or even unilateral (see **Figs. 6** and **7**).[18,25,26] Because cysts can appear at any age, it is generally not suitable to expose the offspring of known carriers of ADPKD to routine sequential sonograms. (2) The glomerulocystic form of ADPKD is mostly seen in fetuses and infants.[14] The kidneys are significantly enlarged, diffusely hyperechoic, and show evidence of discrete subcapsular cysts (see **Figs. 8–10**). In the absence of oligohydramnios, the prognosis is good; in some cases there is a reduction in renal size following birth. (3) In the contiguous genes syndrome (PKD_1 and TSC_2), because the PKD_1 gene is immediately adjacent to the tuberous sclerosis TSC_2 gene on chromosome 16, a large deletion may involve both loci.[27,28] Accordingly, renal US then shows both

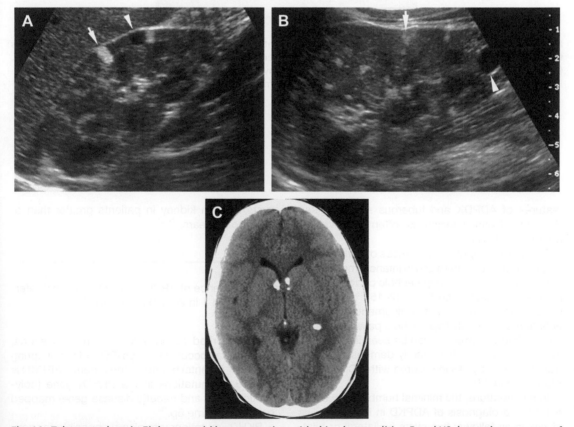

Fig. 11. Tuberous sclerosis. Eight-year-old boy presenting with skin abnormalities. Renal US shows the presence of both angiomyolipomas (*arrows*) and cysts (*arrowheads*) in the right renal cortex (*A*) and the medulla of the left lower kidney (*B*). (*C*) Brain CT shows calcified subependymal nodules classic for tuberous sclerosis.

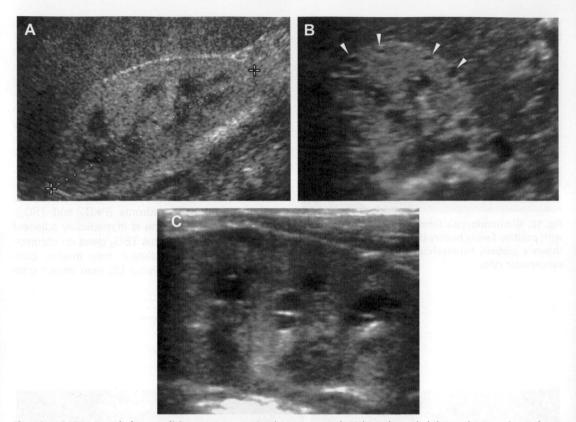

Fig. 12. ADPKD. Renal abnormalities were recognized on antenatal US (not shown). (*A*) Renal US on day 1 shows the right kidney (*cursors*) measures 6 cm; the cortex is hyperechoic but corticomedullary differentiation is present. (*B*) Transverse sonogram of the right kidney at 6 months shows numerous small cysts (*arrowheads*). (*C*) High-resolution US at 1 year of age demonstrating the cortical and medullary location of the small cysts.

features of ADPDK and tuberous sclerosis (see **Fig. 11**). Brain imaging is often positive for tuberous sclerosis.

Other sonographic appearances of ADPKD may be encountered in utero and in infancy: moderately enlarged kidneys with hyperechoic cortex and hypoechoic medulla (see **Figs. 12–15**)[29]; moderate renal enlargement without corticomedullary differentiation and slightly hyperechoic parenchyma; or a completely normal US can be seen in preteens. In my practice, we have rarely demonstrated extrarenal cysts by US in children with ADPKD (see **Figs. 16** and **17**).

In the literature, the minimal number of cysts to establish a diagnosis of ADPKD in PKD_1 families at risk is as follows: two cysts (unilateral or bilateral) between the age of 15 and 29; two cysts in each kidney between the age of 30 and 59; four cysts in each kidney in patients greater than or equal to 60 years.[30,31]

ARPKD

Prevalence
The prevalence of ARPKD is quoted in most references to be 1 in 20,000 live births.[32,33]

Genetics
Being inherited as an autosomal-recessive trait, ARPKD may occur in siblings (25% of the offspring of carrier parents) but not in the parents. ARPKD is caused by mutations in the $PKHD_1$ gene (polycystic kidney and hepatic disease gene) mapped on chromosome 6p.[34]

$PKHD_1$ mutations are also responsible for nonsyndromic congenital hepatic fibrosis and Caroli syndrome. Like the polycystins of ADPKD, the

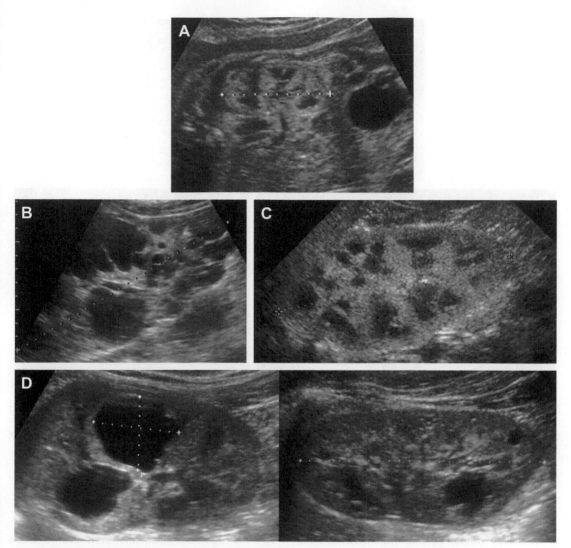

Fig. 13. ADPKD. Case referred for abnormal fetal kidneys. (*A*) Obstetric US at 34 WGA shows echogenic cortex in a kidney with preservation of corticomedullary differentiation. (*B*) Renal US of mother reveals previously unknown ADPKD. (*C*) Neonatal renal US shows a 57-mm long echogenic kidney (*cursors*) with prominent medulla. (*D*) Longitudinal sonogram at 3 years of age shows typical features of ADPKD present in both kidneys.

ARPKD protein, fibrocystin, is localized in primary cilia in the renal tubules.

Pathology

ARPKD affects the kidneys and the liver, with specific histologic involvement of both target organs: cystic dilatation of the renal tubules; biliary dysgenesis and hepatic fibrosis. As a general rule, the phenotype of ARPKD in the kidney and the liver varies in inverse proportions. The form with severe renal involvement is the more common and is

manifested around birth. Conversely, the form with more severe liver impairment and less severe renal damage is less common and usually is manifested later in infancy or childhood. In the perinatal-neonatal form of ARPKD, the kidneys are massively and symmetrically enlarged. Renal enlargement is caused by the fusiform dilatation of all collecting ducts in the medulla and in the cortex.

In later presentation of ARPDK (congenital hepatic fibrosis), the renal involvement consists

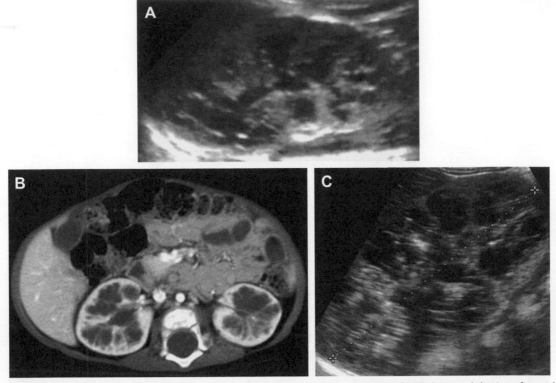

Fig. 14. ADPKD with early predominant medullary involvement. No contributive family history. (*A*) US preformed at 5 months of age for urinary tract infection shows cysts within the medulla. (*B*) Contrast-enhanced CT demonstrates the same medullary hypodensities. Surgical biopsy of the right kidney proved ADPKD. (*C*) US follow-up at 3 years of age shows that multiple cysts have grown in the medullary pyramids (right kidney length = 11 cm).

of medullary ductal ectasia with minimal renal enlargement. The diffuse hepatic lesion is seen in the portal spaces: enlarged, fibrotic portal areas; proliferation and ectasia of bile ducts; and hypoplasia of portal vein branches.

Occasionally, the liver lesion is isolated (Caroli disease). Caroli disease is exceedingly rare in the pediatric age group.

Clinical features and natural history

In the most severe perinatal form, the markedly enlarged kidneys in utero result in oligohydramnios, pulmonary hypoplasia, and Potter sequence. Perinatal survival depends mostly on the degree of pulmonary hypoplasia. Approximately 30% of newborns with renal predominant ARPKD die shortly after birth. In patients who survive the neonatal period, systemic hypertension is seen in approximately 80% of cases; progressive impaired renal function may lead to renal transplantation at a variable age. As children with ARPKD age, complications from liver disease become more significant.[35]

Congenital hepatic fibrosis may result in portal hypertension and also in biliary sepsis. Cholangitis (fever of unknown origin) can be the initial presentation of some ARPKD patients. Hepatocellular function is rarely altered. The kidneys in liver-predominant ARPKD may be normal or slightly enlarged, and may exhibit various degrees of medullary ductal ectasia or macrocystic disease.

Recent series have shown that the prognosis of ARPKD for children who survive the neonatal period and the first months of life is not as dismal as classically considered.

Sonographic features

The US patterns of ARPKD are variable, yet characteristic in most cases, especially when suggestive findings are demonstrated in association in the kidneys and the liver (**Figs. 18–28**).[36–40] High-resolution probes have proved to be very contributive.[41]

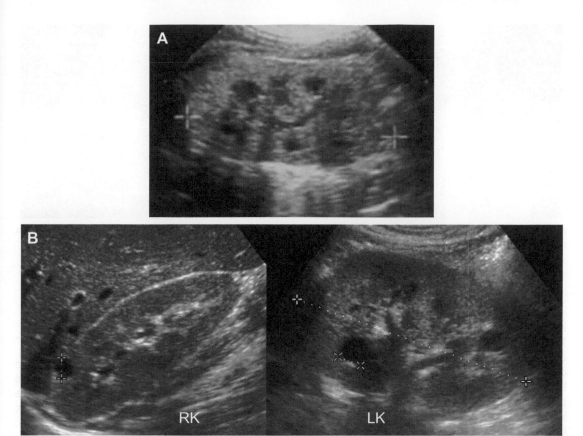

Fig. 15. ADPKD with slow progression on sequential examinations. (*A*) Neonatal US shows a slightly enlarged kidney with echogenic cortex and hypoechoic medulla. (*B*) Follow-up at 15 years of age shows mild changes of ADPKD in both kidneys.

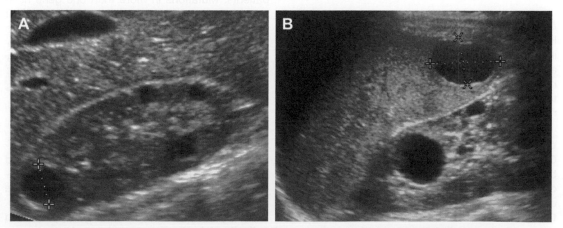

Fig. 16. ADPKD in a 15-year-old patient. (*A*) Renal US shows cysts in the cortex and medulla of the right kidney. (*B*) Image of the left upper quadrant shows a single lower pole splenic cyst (*cursors*), along with cysts in the left kidney.

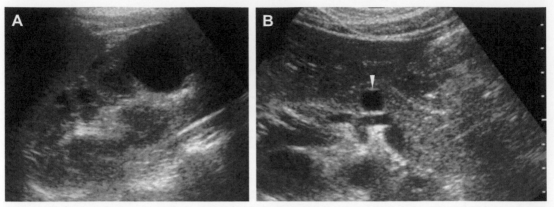

Fig. 17. ADPKD in a 12-year-old patient. (*A*) Longitudinal sonogram of the left kidney shows multiple cysts. (*B*) A single 8-mm cyst (*arrowhead*) is present within the pancreas.

Renal features of ARPKD

Marked bilateral nephromegaly with diffuse hyper-echogenicity of both cortex and medulla, loss of corticomedullary differentiation, poor definition of the collecting system, and preserved contours are seen in utero and around birth. In patients who survive, US shows decreased renal length over time. Moderate, bilateral nephromegaly with hypoechoic outer cortical rim, reversed cortico-medullary differentiation, medullary macrocysts, or echoic nonshadowing dots or foci in medullary location is usually demonstrated in children and teenagers. Both renal sonographic patterns of ARPKD (huge bright kidneys, pseudomedullary nephrocalcinosis in moderately enlarged kidneys) are highly suggestive of the diagnosis. The two patterns can be demonstrated over time in the same patient.

Liver features of ARPKD

Hepatomegaly with left lobe predominance, increased liver echogenicity (periportal thickening), and biliary cysts or focal dilatations are the US hall-marks of congenital hepatic fibrosis. Portal hyper-tension complicating congenital hepatic fibrosis results in splenomegaly and venous collaterals.

Other imaging modalities

CT and MR imaging may be useful in selective cases by displaying nephromegaly; renal tubular cystic dilatation ("striated" appearance, medullary cysts); hepatosplenomegaly; peripheral biliary dila-tations; and cysts. Because of the risk of proce-dure-related cholangitis, percutaneous or retrograde opacification of the biliary tree is contra-indicated in ARPKD patients.

Nephronophthisis

Prevalence

Nephronophthisis (NPH) and medullary cystic disease share the same pathology and clinical features. They differ in their mode of inheritance (autosomal recessive vs autosomal dominant); age of occurrence and of end-stage renal disease; and extrarenal involvement. NPH is an uncommon condition, seen in 1 to 2 per 100,000 live births. It accounts for 10% to 20% of cases of renal failure in childhood.

Genetics

NPH, an autosomal-recessive disorder, is geneti-cally heterogeneous and eight causative genes have been identified.[42] NPHP$_1$ gene mutations on chromosome 2 are found in 50% to 80% of patients. Mutations in more than one gene have been reported. It is also estimated that 15% of new mutations occur in the NPH–medullary cystic disease complex. The NPHP genes encode neph-rocystins localized in primary cilia of renal tubular epithelial cell, and in the photoreceptor cilia (ex-plaining the association of NPH with retinitis pigmentosa).

Pathology

NPH is characterized by a chronic diffuse tubuloin-terstitial nephritis that progresses to fibrosis and terminal renal failure. Small cysts at the corticome-dullary junction or within the medulla become visible late in the course of the disease process. These cysts arise from the distal convoluted and collecting tubules. Tubular basement membranes are characteristically thickened in the juvenile and adolescent forms of NPH.

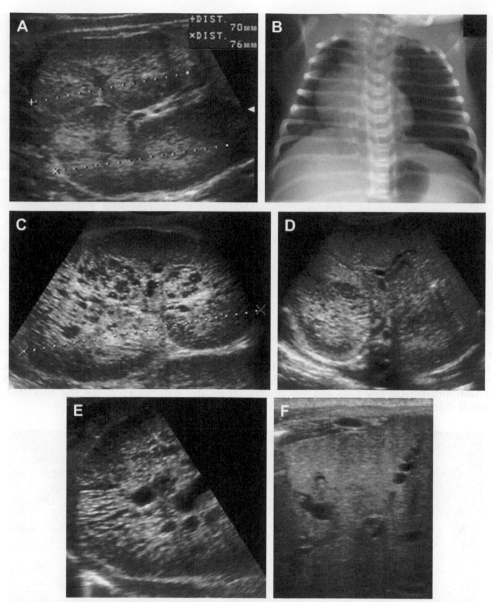

Fig. 18. ARPKD; neonatal form. (*A*) Obstetric US at 30 WGA shows marked bilateral nephromegaly. There was also oligohydramnios and small fetal thorax. (*B*) Chest radiograph at birth shows bilateral pneumothoraces and underlying pulmonary hypoplasia. (*C*) Longitudinal right renal sonogram at birth shows a markedly enlarged kidney (9 cm) with diffuse tubular dilatation in the cortex and medulla. (*D*) Transverse sonogram shows the echogenic right kidney and associated biliary ectasia. (*E*) High-resolution US of the kidney shows multiple dilated renal tubules and medullary cysts. (*F*) High-resolution US of the liver shows tubular ectasia and small parenchymal cysts. Despite aggressive therapy, the patient died at 5 weeks of age.

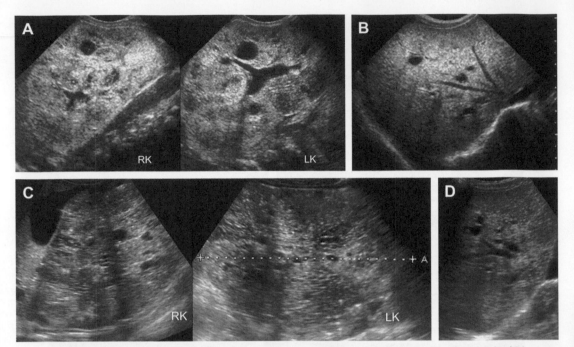

Fig. 19. ARPKD; neonatal form with US follow-up. (*A*) Longitudinal and transverse sonogram of the kidneys on day 2 of life shows bilateral nephromegaly with hyperechogenicity and medullary cysts. (*B*) The liver is mildly echogenic and contains some small cysts. (*C*) At 6 years of age, ultrasound shows enlarged kidneys (19 cm in length) with innumerable tiny cysts and loss of corticomedullary differentiation. (*D*) The associated biliary dysgenesis is characteristic of ARPKD.

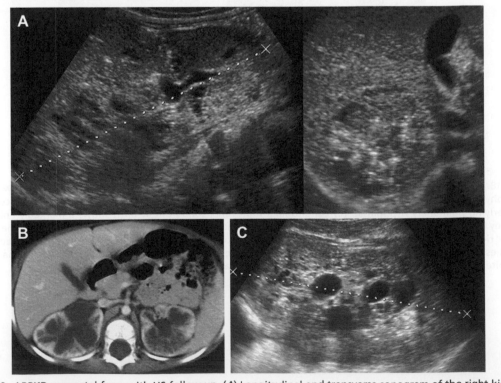

Fig. 20. ARPKD; neonatal form with US follow-up. (*A*) Longitudinal and transverse sonogram of the right kidney at 1.5 years of age shows an enlarged kidney (12 cm) with medullary cystic dilatations and echoic dots. (*B*) Contrast-enhanced CT correlation at the same age. (*C*) Longitudinal renal sonogram at 8 years of age shows that the medullary macrocysts are more obvious within a 16-cm long kidney.

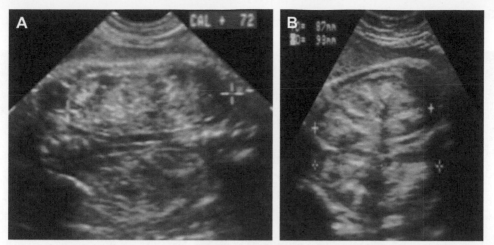

Fig. 21. ARPKD; changing patterns during pregnancy. (*A*) Obstetric US at 30 WGA shows that both kidneys are significantly enlarged and hyperechoic. (*B*) Obstetric US at 36 WGA in the same patient. There is now evidence of a peripheral hypoechoic rim with marked medullary hyperechogenicity.

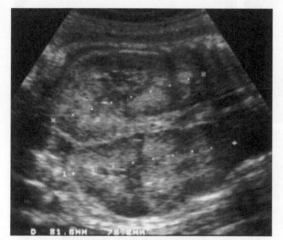

Fig. 22. ARPKD; third trimester US. Both kidneys measure 8 cm and have a peripheral hypoechoic rim surrounding hyperechoic parenchyma.

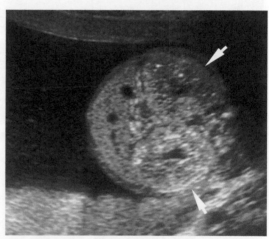

Fig. 23. Early severe fetal ARPDK. Obstetric US at 19 WGA shows large dedifferentiated kidneys fill more than 50% of the fetal abdomen. The parents elected to terminate the pregnancy. Pathology was consistent with ARPKD.

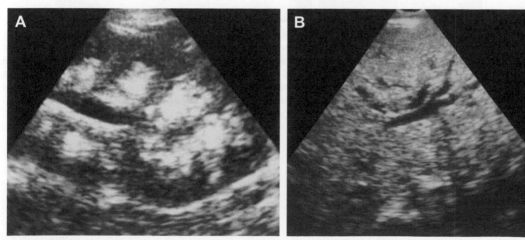

Fig. 24. ARPKD; medullary pattern in a 2-year-old girl. (*A*) Renal US shows a strikingly hyperechoic medulla (pseudonephrocalcinosis) in a moderately enlarged kidney. (*B*) The liver is hyperechoic with biliary ectasia.

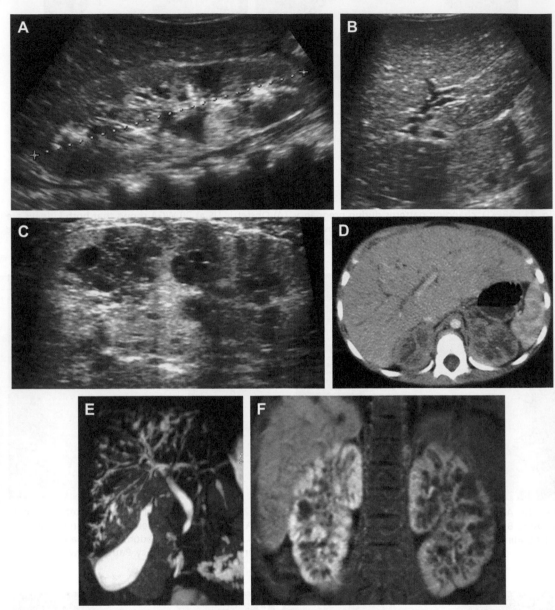

Fig. 25. ARPKD; 2 year old investigated for fever of unknown origin. Imaging correlations (US, CT, MRI) showing the coexisting renal and hepatic lesions of ARPKD. Liver biopsy grew *Escherichia coli*. (*A*) Longitudinal sonogram of the right kidney shows an elongated echogenic kidney. (*B*) US of the liver shows diffusely echogenic and coarse parenchyma with biliary ectasia. (*C*) High-resolution US of the kidney shows numerous small medullary cysts. (*D*) Contrast-enhanced CT shows hepatic biliary ectasia and poorly enhancing renal cortex. (*E*) Coronal T2-weighted MRI shows striking ectasia of the biliary system. (*F*) Contrast-enhanced coronal T1-weighted MRI shows innumerable small medullary renal cysts and architectural distortion.

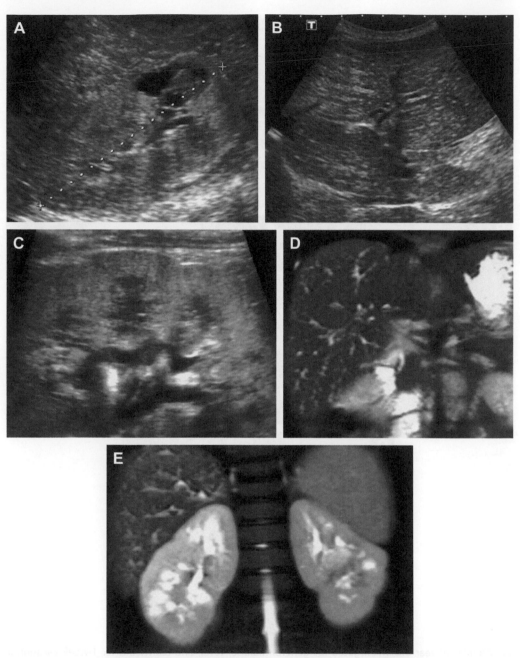

Fig. 26. ARPKD; 18 month old with fever of unknown origin of several weeks duration. Liver biopsy grew *E coli*. (*A*) Longitudinal right renal sonogram shows an echogenic kidney with poor corticomedullary differentiation and lower pole cortical and medullary cysts. (*B*) US of the liver shows diffusely echogenic and coarse parenchyma with biliary ectasia. (*C*) High-resolution renal US shows subtle medullary cystic changes. (*D*) Coronal T2-weighted MRI shows ectasia of the biliary system. (*E*) Coronal T2-weighted MRI shows medullary renal cysts.

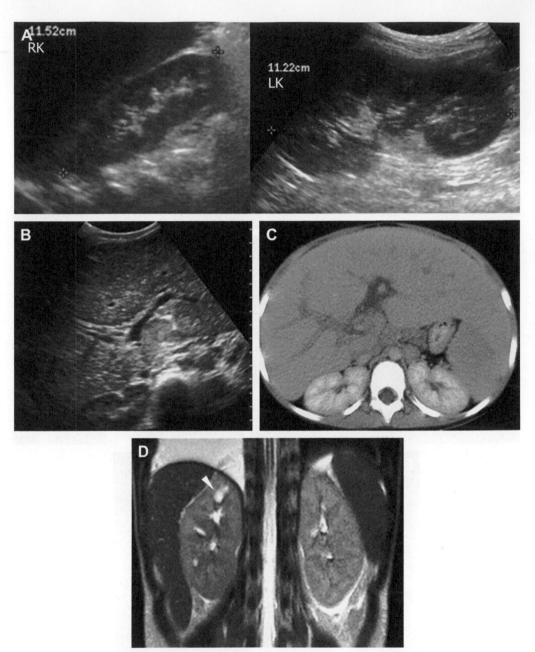

Fig. 27. ARPKD; 10 year old investigated for general malaise, fever, and diarrhea after 1-week vacation in the Dominican Republic. Liver biopsy specimen grew *Salmonella*. (*A*) Renal US shows slightly enlarged kidneys. No cysts or abnormality of parenchymal echostructure are seen. (*B*) The liver is enlarged and hyperechoic with minimal biliary ectasia. (*C*) Contrast-enhanced CT shows hepatomegaly and biliary ectasia; the kidneys appear normal. (*D*) Coronal T2-weighted MRI shows a medullary cyst (*arrowhead*) in the upper pole of the right kidney.

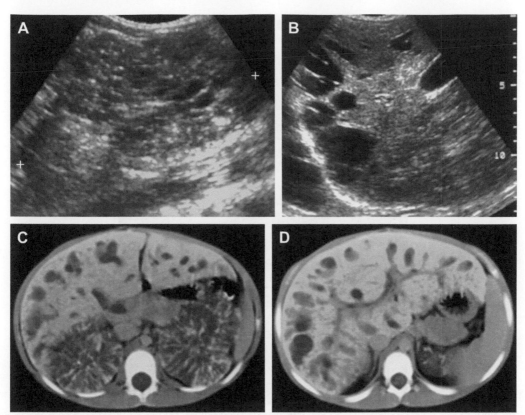

Fig. 28. ARPKD; 9 year old with severe involvement of both the kidneys and the liver. (*A*) Longitudinal sonogram of the enlarged left kidney (*cursors*) shows cystic and hyperechoic changes throughout the parenchyma. (*B*) Liver US shows biliary ectasia and peripheral biliary cysts. (*C*) Contrast-enhanced CT shows enlarged kidneys with a striated tubular nephrogram. (*D*) Contrast-enhanced CT of the liver shows biliary cysts that correlated with the US findings. There is no evidence of portal hypertension (normal spleen size).

Clinical features and natural history

The onset of the disease is insidious. The concentration tubular impairment causes polyuria and polydipsia, the usual presenting symptoms of NPH. Progression to end-stage renal failure occurs at different ages, depending on the form of NPH. In the juvenile form of NPH, the most frequent, caused by mutations in NPHP$_1$, polyuria and polydipsia start at 4 to 6 years of age and end-stage renal disease occurs at 13 years (median age). In the infantile and adolescent forms of NPH, renal failure occurs at 1 to 3 years and 19 years, respectively.

Extrarenal involvement (ocular, neurologic, skeletal, hepatic) is seen in 20% of cases of NPH, and some syndromes feature NPH or are associated with NPHP genes mutations (**Box 2**).

Medullary cystic disease, an autosomal-dominant condition, differs from NPH by a later age of occurrence of uremia (in adulthood) and the absence of extrarenal association (except for gout).

Sonographic features

US may be normal early in the disease (**Figs. 29–31**). Loss of corticomedullary differentiation and

---

Box 2

Syndromes associated with NPHP genes mutations

- Senior-Loken → retinitis pigmentosa
- Cogan → ocular motor apraxia
- Joubert type B → vermis hypoplasia
- Saldino-Mainzer → cone-shaped epiphysis
- Sensenbrenner → cranioectodermal dysplasia
- Jeune → short ribs
- Rhyns → hypopituitarism, retinitis pigmentosa, skeletal dysplasia
- Boichis → biliary duct proliferation and liver fibrosis
- Alstrom → retinal dystrophy, hearing loss, obesity, type 2 diabetes mellitus
- Meckel-Gruber → encephalocele, polydactyly, cystic kidneys

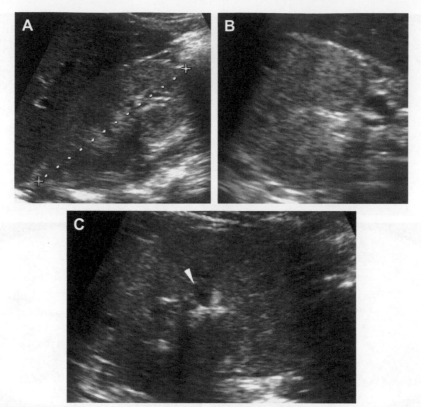

Fig. 29. NPH; Cogan syndrome in a 12 year old with chronic renal failure. (*A*) Longitudinal sonogram shows right kidney (*cursors*) measures 9.4 cm, with complete disappearance of the corticomedullary differentiation and hyperechoic cortex. (*B*) Transverse image of the right kidney shows a small cyst at the corticomedullary junction. (*C*) Longitudinal sonogram of the left kidney also shows a medullary cyst (*arrowhead*).

parenchymal hyperechogenicity are often observed in normal-sized kidneys. Renal cysts (medullary or corticomedullary in location) become visible when patients have progressed to end-stage renal failure. Approximately 25% of patients have no grossly visible cysts at pathology or at US. The most suggestive US pattern in NPH before dialysis is made of few medullary cysts in dedifferentiated kidneys of almost normal size (an uncommon occurrence in end-stage kidneys).[43–45]

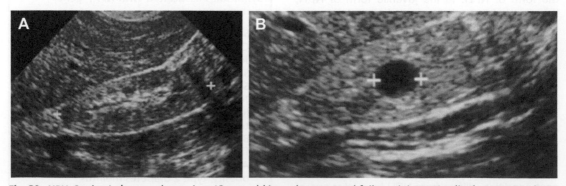

Fig. 30. NPH; Senior-Loken syndrome in a 12 year old in end-stage renal failure. (*A*) Longitudinal sonogram shows the right kidney (*cursors*) measures 8 cm, with loss of corticomedullary differentiation. (*B*) A single discrete medullary cyst (*cursors*) is seen in the right kidney.

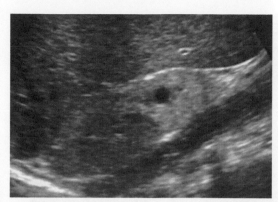

Fig. 31. NPH; 10-year-old prerenal transplantation. Longitudinal sonogram of the right kidney showing a single medullary cyst within a hyperechoic kidney.

Box 3
Malformation syndromes with renal cysts

- Tuberous sclerosis
- Bardet-Biedl
- Beckwith-Wiedemann
- Meckel-Gruber
- von Hippel-Lindau
- Zellweger
- Short ribs polydactyly
- Jeune
- Ellis-van Creveld
- Orofaciodigital type I
- Glutaric aciduria type II
- Ivemark (renal-hepatic-pancreatic dysplasia)
- Marden-Walker
- VACTERL
- Smith-Lemli-Opitz
- Alagille
- Ehler-Danlos
- Turner
- Trisomies (13–15, 18, 21, 10)

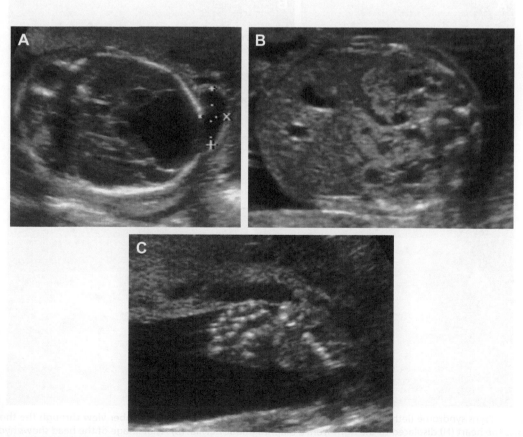

Fig. 32. Meckel-Gruber syndrome (lethal). Obstetric US at 19 WGA. (*A*) Abnormal posterior fossa with cephalocele (*cursors*). (*B*) Bilateral renal cystic medullary abnormalities. (*C*) Polydactyly.

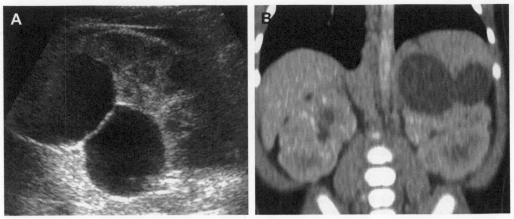

Fig. 33. Beckwith-Wiedemann syndrome in a 14-day-old infant. (*A*) Longitudinal renal sonogram showing macrocysts in the left kidney. (*B*) Reformatted coronal CT shows large cysts in the upper pole of the left kidney.

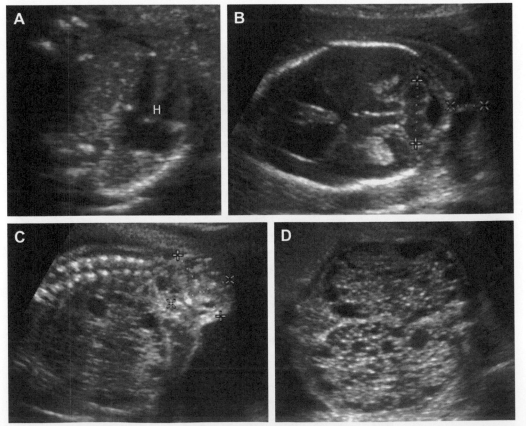

Fig. 34. Fryns syndrome (lethal). Obstetric US at 19 WGA. (*A*) Transverse four-chamber view through the thorax shows the heart (H) displaced to the right from a diaphragmatic hernia. (*B*) Axial image of the head shows hydrocephalus and a nuchal cystic hygroma. (*C*) Longitudinal view of the distal spine shows a sacrococcygeal teratoma (*cursors*). (*D*) Both kidneys are enlarged with diffuse severe cystic changes.

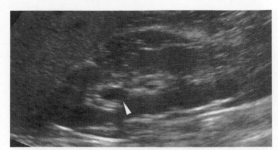

Fig. 35. Bardet-Biedl syndrome. Longitudinal renal sonogram in a 10 year old shows loss of corticomedullary differentiation. A single medullary cyst (*arrowhead*) is apparent.

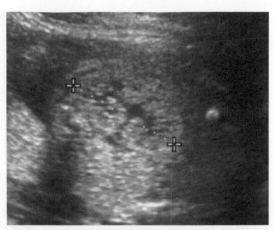

Fig. 36. Bardet-Biedl syndrome; prenatal diagnosis. Obstetric US at 21 WGA shows an enlarged 4-cm abnormally echogenic kidney. Polydactyly was also demonstrated (not shown). Parents elected to terminate the pregnancy.

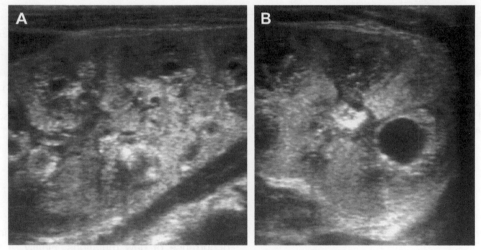

Fig. 37. Three day old with abnormal chromosome 10. High-resolution US of the right kidney (*A*) and left kidney (*B*) shows the extensive medullary cystic changes.

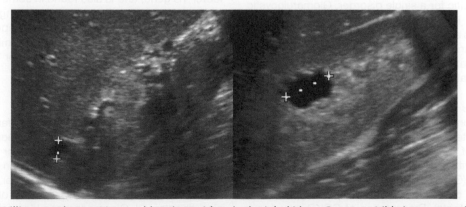

Fig. 38. Williams syndrome; 14-year-old patient with a single right kidney. Cysts are visible in cortex and medulla (*cursors*).

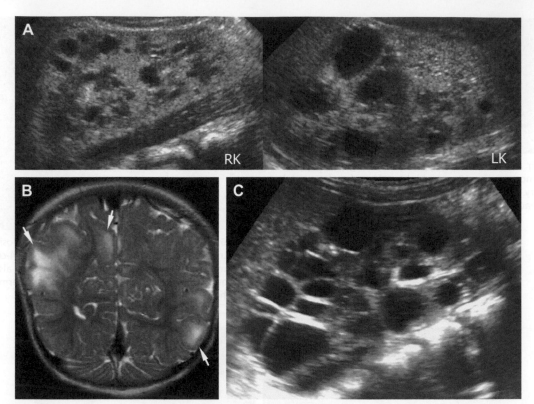

Fig. 39. Tuberous sclerosis. Postnatal investigation of bilateral renal cysts seen in utero. (*A*) Renal US at 1 month of age shows bilateral cysts are present, both in the cortex and medulla. (*B*) Brain MRI at 10 months of age. Coronal T2-weighted image shows bilateral subcortical hamartomas (*arrows*) characteristic of tuberous sclerosis. (*C*) Renal US at 2 years of age shows progression of the cysts.

Glomerulocystic Kidney Disease

Nosology

Glomerulocystic refers to a glomerular cyst (distended Bowman spaces). Glomerular cysts are not specific for a single disorder. Glomerulocystic disease is a primary disease; glomerulocystic kidney is a kidney with glomerular cysts as a dominant manifestation but of diverse etiologies (eg, malformation syndromes, such as tuberous sclerosis, oral-facial-digital syndrome type I).[46–48]

Genetics

Most glomerulocystic kidney diseases (GCKD) are transmitted according to an autosomal-dominant mode of inheritance and discovered in infants either within the context of a familial history of ADPKD (GCKD of young infants in ADPKD phenotype) or outside this context (sporadic GCKD of young infants). Presentation of GCKD may occur in older children and adults, both of familial (dominant) and sporadic types, reflecting the occurrence of new mutations. Finally, a familial hypoplastic in short, GCKD has been described in relation to mutations of the hepatocyte nuclear factor 1B gene, and is also found in some families with maturity-onset diabetes of the young type 5. Genital tract malformations are also reported in HNF1B mutations. GCKD is either dominant or sporadic and occurs either in infants or in older patients.

Sonographic features

In the GCKD variant of ADPKD in infants, the kidneys are enlarged, hyperechoic, without corticomedullary differentiation. Subcapsular cortical cysts are fairly typical of GCKD. Cysts can develop prenatally or only after birth. In the other form of GCKD, the kidneys may be hypoplastic, of normal size, or enlarged. Glomerulocystic kidneys are addressed with the malformation syndromes.

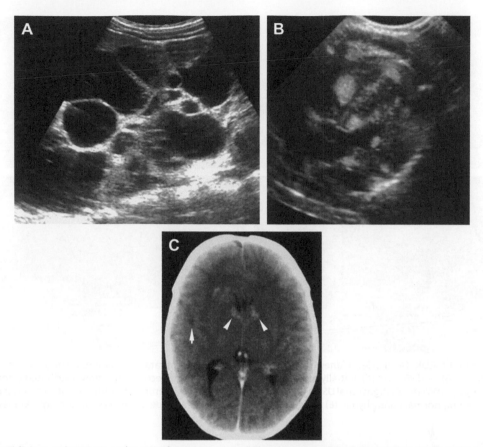

Fig. 40. Tuberous sclerosis complex. Newborn investigated because prenatal US had shown cardiac rhabdomyomas and renal cysts. (*A*) Longitudinal sonogram of the right kidney shows extensive cystic change. The left kidney appeared similar. (*B*) Multiple echogenic cardiac rhabdomyomas are easily seen. (*C*) Contrast-enhanced CT of the brain shows subcortical hamartomas and enhancing lesions at the foramina of Monro typical of tuberous sclerosis.

Malformation Syndromes

Nosology and genetics

Numerous syndromes can present with renal cysts (**Box 3**).[14,49–54] They can be subdivided according to (1) their mode of inheritance (autosomal dominant [eg, tuberous sclerosis, von Hippel-Lindau disease], autosomal recessive [eg, Meckel-Gruber, Jeune, Bardet-Biedl], X-linked dominant [oral-facial-digital syndrome type I], chromosome disorders [trisomies D, E, 21, Turner]); (2) their pathologic characteristics: diffuse cystic dysplasia as in Meckel-Gruber, Beckwith-Wiedemann, glutaric aciduria type II, VACTERL, glomerulocystic kidneys as in tuberous sclerosis, oral-facial-digital syndrome type I, short ribs polydactyly, Jeune, Zellweger, trisomy 13; and (3) their associated manifestations and clinical course: some syndromes are lethal in utero (eg, Meckel-Gruber (**Fig. 32**), oral-facial-digital

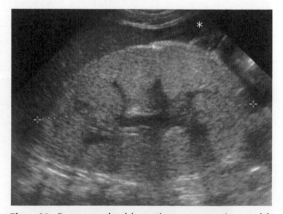

Fig. 41. Four-month-old patient presenting with rapidly evolving nephrotic syndrome. Renal sonogram shows a large (7.5 cm) echoic kidney (*cursors*) with loss of corticomedullary differentiation and coexistent ascites (*asterisk*). Peritoneal dialysis was initiated at 8 months of age, followed by successful renal transplantation.

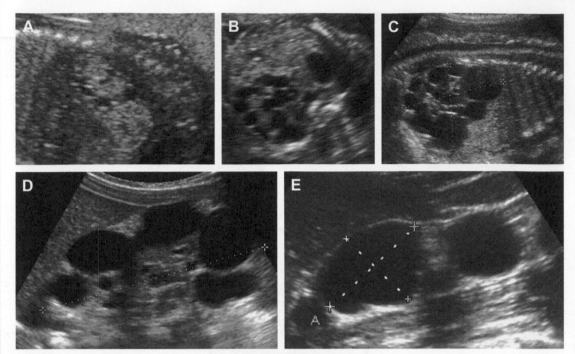

Fig. 42. Right MCDK. Normal left kidney (not shown). Prenatal and postnatal correlation. Obstetric US at 16 WGA (*A*), 20 WGA (*B*), and 30 WGA (*C*). Initially peripheral at 16 WGA, the cysts become randomly distributed throughout the kidney by 30 WGA. (*D*) Right renal US on day 5 of life shows cysts of different size with thin intervening septa and no intervening normal parenchyma. (*E*) Renal US at 4 years of age shows persisting cysts in the right kidney.

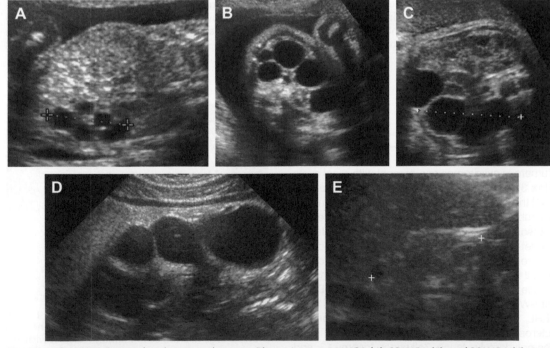

Fig. 43. Left MCDK. Prenatal and postnatal course. Obstetric US at 21 WGA (*A*), 32 WGA (*B*), and 36 WGA (*C*). Renal macrocysts are seen throughout pregnancy. (*D*) Renal US at 1 month of age shows the left kidney measures 7 cm and shows the multiple cysts, without evidence of a dilated pelvis. The right kidney was normal (not shown). (*E*) Left renal US at 2 years of age shows and atrophic kidney (4.5 cm) (*cursors*) with near complete resolution of the cysts.

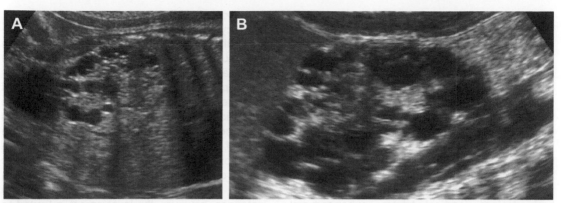

Fig. 44. Peripheral cystic pattern of MCDK. (*A*) Obstetric US at 33 WGA shows multiple peripheral cysts are seen in the right kidney. (*B*) Renal US on day 15 of life shows that most cysts are peripheral in location. The left kidney was normal (not shown).

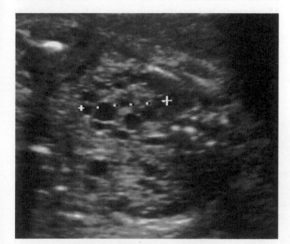

Fig. 45. Bilateral fetal MCDK (lethal form). Obstetric US at 20 WGA shows bilateral peripheral cystic involvement. There was no visible bladder and severe oligohydramnios.

syndrome type I in boys), some can be overlooked in childhood and diagnosed only later in life (eg, Bardet-Biedl syndrome, characterized by pigmentary retinopathy, distal limb anomalies, renal anomalies, obesity, hypogenitalism in males, mental retardation), some are manifested clinically only in adulthood but can be diagnosed by mutation analysis (presymptomatic test) in family members (eg, von Hippel-Lindau disease).

The presence of associated malformations (polydactyly, central nervous system anomaly, overgrowth, small chest, cardiac malformations, and so forth) may suggest the diagnosis (eg, polydactyly in association with renal cysts is seen in Meckel-Gruber, Bardet-Biedl, short ribs polydactyly, Simpson-Golabi-Behmel). Among the various malformation syndromes (**Figs. 33–38**), cystic kidneys of tuberous sclerosis are important to consider distinctly (**Figs. 39 and 40**).[55–58]

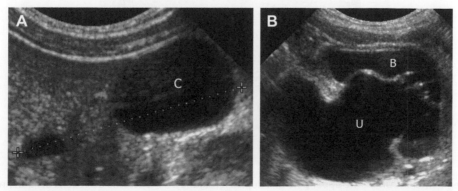

Fig. 46. Hypodysplastic right kidney with coexisting ureterocele. (*A*) The right kidney measures 3.5 cm in length with a lower pole macrocyst (C). (*B*) An ipsilateral ureterocele (U) is seen within the bladder (B).

Genetics, prevalence, and nosology

Tuberous sclerosis complex (TSC) is an auto-somal-dominant syndrome linked to TSC_1 and TSC_2 genes, located respectively on chromosomes 9p and 16p. TSC affects 1 in 6000 live births. Renal cysts in TSC may be associated with both TSC_1 and TSC_2 mutations, without or with coexisting deletion of PKD_1 gene (adjacent genes syndrome).[27,28]

TSC is diagnosed based on major and minor features. The major features include facial angiofibromas; ungual fibromas; hypomelanotic macules; shagreen patches; retinal hamartomas; brain lesions (cortical tubers, subependymal nodules, astrocytomas); cardiac rhabdomyomas; lymphangiomyomatosis; and renal angiomyolipomas. Minor features are enamel dental pits, rectal polyps, bone cysts, gingival fibromas, nonrenal hamartomas, renal cysts, and renal carcinomas. A definite diagnosis of TSC now requires two or more distinct types of lesions. The disease tends to be more severe in patients with TSC_2 mutations.

Sonographic features

Renal cysts occur either exclusively or in association with angiomyolipomas. Cysts are variable in size, number, and location, involving both the cortex and the medulla of the kidney. The classic cystic pattern of TSC may also be associated with the glomerulocystic kidney pattern. In one pediatric series of TSC cases,[55] renal cysts occurred in 47% of cases, angiomyolipomas in 80% of cases, and cysts associated with angiomyolipomas in 25% of cases. In most pediatric cases of TSC with renal cysts, neuroimaging shows suggestive brain lesions. In some instances, however, the involvement is limited to the kidney.

Microcystic Kidney Disease

Microcystic kidney disease refers to the congenital nephrotic syndrome of the Finnish type. The prevalence of the congenital nephrotic syndrome is 1

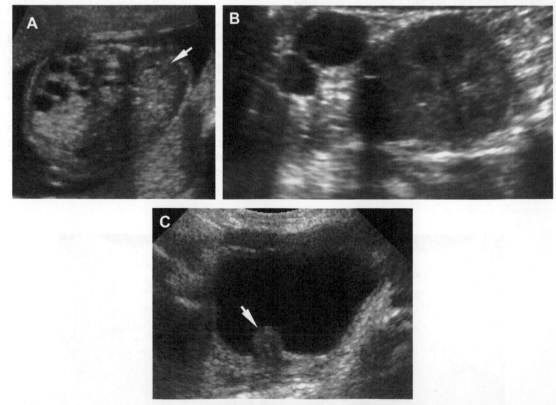

Fig. 47. Segmental MCDK on the upper pole of a duplex left kidney. (*A*) Obstetric US at 20 WGA showing the left multicystic dysplasia. The right kidney (*arrow*) is normal. (*B*) Left renal US on day 10 of life shows dysplastic cysts in the upper pole and normal lower pole. (*C*) A small collapsed ureterocele (*arrow*) is seen in the bladder.

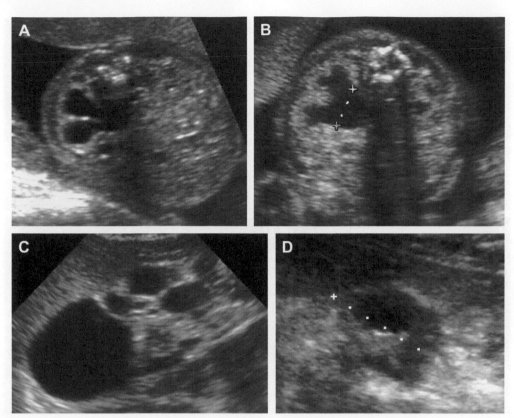

Fig. 48. Hydronephrotic form of MCDK. Obstetric US at 21 WGA (*A*) and 27 WGA (*B*) displaying a pattern suggestive of right kidney ureteropelvic junction obstruction, with hyperechoic renal cortex. (*C*) Right renal US at 1
month of age shows a characteristic pattern of MCDK. Normal left kidney (not shown). (*D*) At 1 year of age, there
is almost complete involution of the dysplastic right kidney (*cursors*).

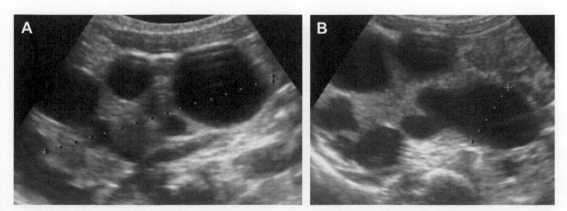

Fig. 49. Intermediate pattern MCDK–ureteropelvic junction obstruction. (*A*) Longitudinal sonogram of right
kidney on day 2 of life shows typical findings of MCDK. (*B*) Transverse sonogram shows a dilated renal pelvis
(*cursors*) without communication with the more peripheral cysts.

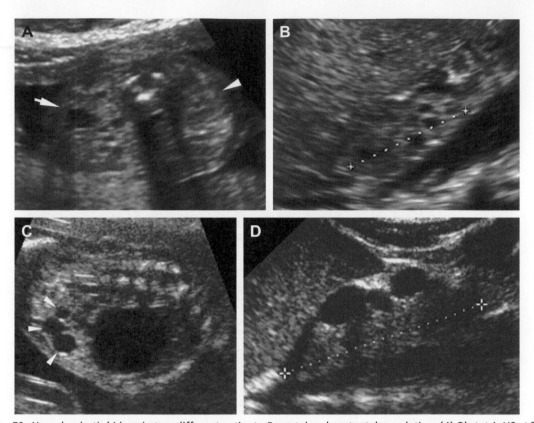

Fig. 50. Hypodysplastic kidney in two different patients. Prenatal and postnatal correlation. (*A*) Obstetric US at 21 WGA (transverse scan). Normal left kidney (*arrowhead*). Dysplastic right kidney (*arrow*). (*B*) Renal US on day 18 in same patient. The dysplastic right kidney (*cursors*) measures 21 mm, the normal left kidney (not shown) measured 47 mm. (*C*) Obstetric US at 20 WGA in second patient. Three cysts (*arrowheads*) are identified in the right kidney. (*D*) Renal US at 1 month of age in second. The hypodysplastic right kidney (*cursors*) measures 3 cm, the normal left kidney (not shown) measured 7.1 cm (compensatory hypertrophy).

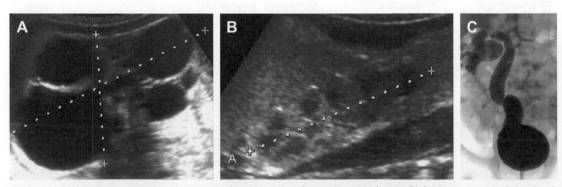

Fig. 51. Left MCDK associated with major right VUR. (*A*) Left renal US on day 5 of life shows a typical dysplastic kidney. (*B*) Longitudinal sonogram of the right kidney (*cursors*) shows slight atrophy but no collecting system dilatation. Intermittent dilatation of the distal right ureter was noted. (*C*) Voiding cystourethrogram (VCUG) shows right grade V VUR.

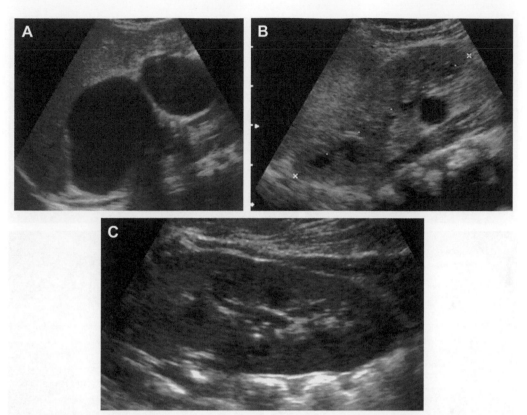

Fig. 52. Right MCKD associated with left renal cysts. (*A*) Right renal US at 4 months of age shows dysplasia with two macrocysts that persisted unchanged on subsequent examinations (up to 6 years of age). (*B*) Three renal cysts were documented within an otherwise normal left kidney (*cursors*). (*C*) At 2 years of age, the renal cysts have resolved and the left kidney is completely normal.

per 10,000 live births in Finland, much less frequent in the non-Finnish population.

An autosomal-recessive inherited disorder, microcystic kidney disease is characterized pathologically by cystic dilatation of proximal and distal tubules. The $NPHS_1$ gene of the disease is mapped on the long arm of chromosome 19.

Sonographically, the kidneys are usually of normal size in utero and at birth, and become markedly enlarged with loss of corticomedullary differentiation subsequently (**Fig. 41**).[59]

Renal Cystic Dysplasia

Pathology

Dysplastic kidneys refer to an abnormal renal development with poorly differentiated nephrons; poorly branched and differentiated collecting ducts ("primitive" tubules); increased stroma; and occasionally parenchymal cysts and metaplastic cartilage.

Physiopathology of renal dysplasia

Normal development of the kidney results from the mutual induction of metanephric blastema and ureteral bud ampullae. Nephron differentiation

---

Box 4
Hyperechoic fetal kidneys

- Coexisting with urinary tract dilatation: ORD (with or without macrocysts)
- Associated with marked nephromegaly: ARPKD
- Coexisting with macrocysts: MCDK, syndromes, (ADPKD)
- Coexisting with associated anomalies: syndromes, trisomies
- Coexisting with macrosomia: overgrowth syndromes (Beckwith-Wiedemann, Perlman, Simpson-Golabi-Behmel, Elejalde)
- Miscellaneous: vascular, tumoral, metabolic causes
- Normal variant

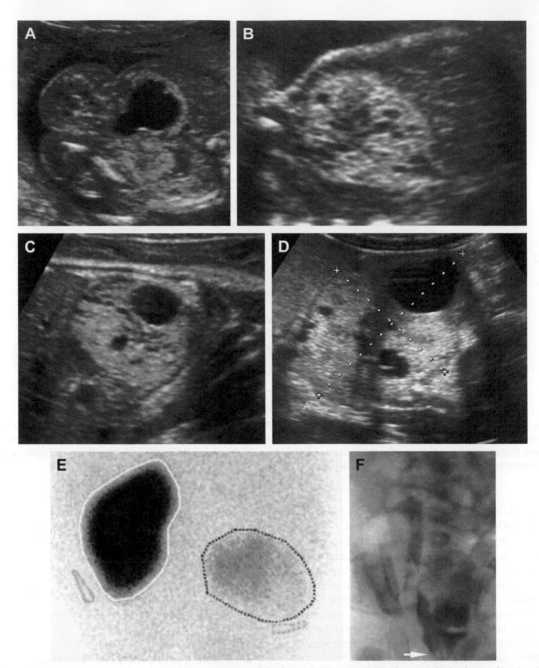

Fig. 53. Right ORD caused by an ectopic megaureter. (*A*) Obstetric US at 18 WGA shows right hydronephrosis with hyperechoic renal cortex. The left kidney was normal (not shown). (*B*) Obstetric US at 23 WGA shows small parenchymal cysts are now visible in the hyperechoic right kidney. (*C*) Obstetric US at 31 WGA shows progression of the cystic dysplasia. (*D*) Right renal US on day 14 shows an enlarged hyperechoic right kidney with macrocysts. Normal left kidney (not shown). (*E*) Scintigraphy shows almost no function of the right kidney. (*F*) VCUG shows the right megaureter inserting ectopically (*arrow*) into the vagina.

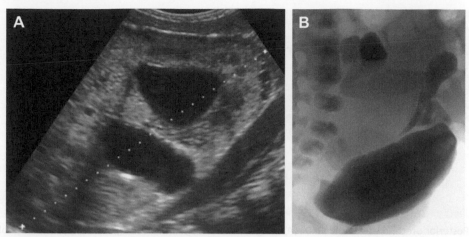

Fig. 54. Right duplex kidney and megaureter detected prenatally. (*A*) US on day 9 of life shows a duplex right kidney with megaureter (not shown) of the upper moiety and peripheral cortical cysts in a diffusely hyperechoic kidney. Normal left kidney (not shown). (*B*) VCUG shows lower pole VUR.

begins at 7 weeks gestational age; the ureteral bud dilates and divides dichotomously to form the renal pelvis, infundibula, calyces, and collecting tubules. Aberrant inductive interactions between epithelial cells of the ureteral bud and mesenchymal cells of the metanephros lead to dysplasia. As a general rule, renal dysplasia results from in utero urinary tract obstruction and ampullary dysfunction.[60,61] The severity of dysplasia depends on the timing, location, and degree of obstruction.[62] Most renal cystic dysplasias occur as sporadic events. Recent advances in the genetics of dysplasia have pointed out, however, that around 10% of cases may have a family history of urinary tract malformations and several genes have been implicated in various congenital abnormalities of the kidney and urinary tract (eg, the TCF_2 gene encoding HNF1B).[63–65]

Multicystic Dysplastic Kidney

Multicystic dysplastic kidney (MCDK) is the most common abdominal mass in newborns after hydronephrosis (**Figs. 42–52**). At the present time, MCDK is most often diagnosed in utero (from 16 weeks gestational age to the third trimester).[66–69] Because of the trend of MCKD to involute prenatally and postnatally, the prevalence of unilateral MCDK is higher in the fetus (1 in 1000–1 in 2000) than in the newborn (1 in 4000).

Bilateral MCDK results in oligohydramnios and the Potter sequence and is lethal. There is a 30% risk of contralateral renal anomaly (ureteropelvic junction obstruction, vesicoureteral reflux, hypoplasia) in unilateral MCDK.

Differentiation of MCDK from hydronephrosis in the fetus and newborn is paramount because of their different management and treatment. Sonographically, MCDK appears as noncommunicating

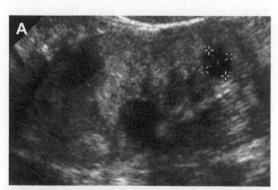

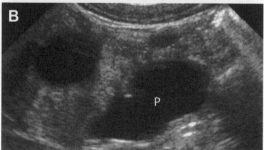

Fig. 55. ORD; 29-day-old infant with palpable left kidney. (*A*) Longitudinal sonogram shows a dysplastic left kidney with peripheral cysts (*cursors*). (*B*) More medial image shows dilatation of the renal pelvis (P). Scintigraphy showed no left renal function. The US pattern is suggestive of an hydronephrotic form of MCDK.

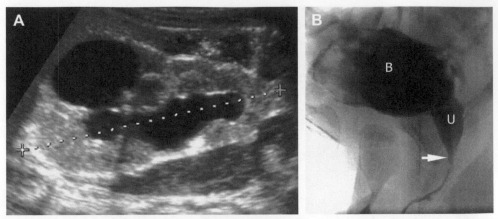

Fig. 56. Posterior urethral valves and ORD. (*A*) Longitudinal sonogram of the right kidney in a 2 week old shows mild hydronephrosis and a large cortical cyst. (*B*) VCUG shows a trabeculated bladder (B) and a dilated posterior urethra (U) narrowing at the partially obstructing valve (*arrow*).

cysts of varying size and shape, within an echogenic renal parenchyma or with well-defined intercystic septa; the larger cyst is not anteromedially located (ie, different from the enlarged pelvis in cases of ureteropelvic junction obstruction); and there is no identifiable renal sinus. The cysts are randomly distributed throughout the kidney with no intervening normal renal parenchyma. Color Doppler ultrasound displays an absent or extremely hypoplastic renal artery. In cases of duplex kidneys, MCDK of the upper pole moiety is sometimes referred to as "segmental cystic dysplasia."[70]

The natural history of MCDK has been clarified by serial sonograms[71–75] on patients managed conservatively: 67% decrease in size, 19% show no change, and 10% increase in size. Involuted MCDK may mimic renal agenesis. There have been rare reports of Wilms tumor and renal cell carcinoma arising in MCDK: this very low frequency of subsequent malignancies has not changed the conservative management of most children with MCDK.[68,69] Sequential sonograms show that 33% of MCDK have completely involuted at 2 years of age, 47% at 5 years, and 59% at 10 years.

Obstructive Renal Dysplasia

Nosology

In obstructive renal dysplasia (ORD), the abnormally developed kidney is caused by fetal urinary obstruction or reflux.[62] In mild ORD, associated with partial lower tract obstruction, the kidney may be of normal size with preserved

corticomedullary differentiation, or diffusely hyperechoic with small subcortical cysts, megacystis, and dilated ureters. Severe ORD with complete lower tract obstruction (urethral atresia) is characterized by marked cystic dysplasia with corticomedullary differentiation effacement. Segmental ORD, associated with duplex kidneys, is typically confined to the upper moiety.

ORD can also be seen in prune-belly syndrome, a male multisystem complex. Prune-belly syndrome features a distended abdomen with redundant skin and defective abdominal wall

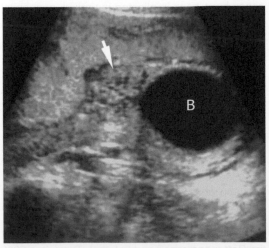

Fig. 57. Prenatal ORD from urethral atresia. Obstetric US shows an enlarged bladder (B) coexisting with extremely dysplastic kidneys (*arrow*), severe oligohydramnios, and small chest.

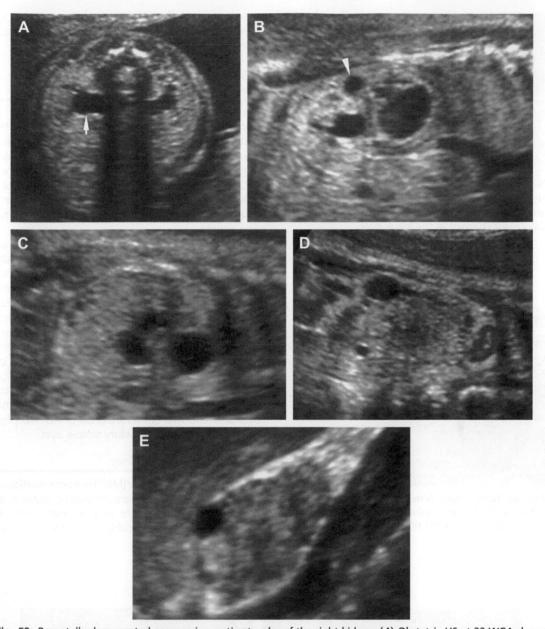

Fig. 58. Prenatally documented progressive cystic atrophy of the right kidney. (*A*) Obstetric US at 22 WGA shows slight dilatation of right kidney pelvis (6 mm, *arrow*). (*B*) Obstetric US at 25 WGA shows right kidney cysts (*arrowhead*) are now visible. (*C*) Obstetric US at 29 WGA shows progression of dysplastic changes in the right kidney. (*D*) Obstetric US at 35 WGA shows atrophy of the dysplastic right kidney. (*E*) Renal sonogram at birth shows a small atrophic cystic right kidney. The left kidney was normal (6 cm, not shown). There was no VUR.

musculature, accompanied by megacystis, mega-ureters, hydronephrotic dysplastic kidneys, and bilateral cryptorchidism.

Sonographic features

The classic antenatal presentation of dysplastic kidneys at sonography is of large bright kidneys with or without cystic spaces (**Box 4**). Serial sonograms may document the delayed visibility of renal cysts within a previously hyperechoic parenchyma (**Figs. 53–58**).

Uniformly echogenic fetal kidneys without visible macrocysts are not uncommon on routine obstetric US, and it is essential to differentiate a normal variant (normal size kidneys, moderately bright cortex, visible corticomedullary

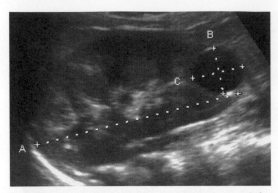

Fig. 59. Simple cyst. One year old investigated for urinary tract infection. Left renal US showed a single simple cyst (*cursors*) at the lower pole.

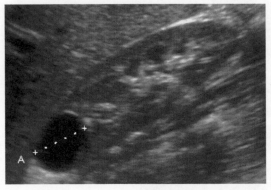

Fig. 60. Simple cyst. Nine year old evaluated for appendicitis. A simple renal cyst (*cursors*) was seen at the upper pole of the right kidney.

differentiation after 20 weeks gestational age, normal bladder, normal amount of amniotic fluid) from a significant renal disease.[76]

NONGENETIC, NONDYSPLASTIC CYSTS
Simple Cysts

Prevalence
Renal simple cysts are seen in around 5% of the general population of any age undergoing abdominal US,[77] and arise in nondiseased kidneys (**Figs. 59–63**). The incidence increases with age: 0.22% in children,[78] up to 20% in 40-year-old patients, and in 33% of individuals after 60 years. A similar prevalence has been noted in all pediatric age groups.

In infants and children, simple cysts appear as solitary lesions. Those detected prenatally commonly resolve before birth.[79] Most renal simple cysts in children remain unchanged on follow-up (74%),[78] and are managed conservatively. The widespread use of US in pediatrics accounts for the detection of renal simple cysts in patients either routinely imaged for a frequent clinical situation (eg, urinary tract infection) or routinely followed after previously treated malignancies. Sonographic follow-up is suggested by most authors to document the stability of the cyst size and rule out a rare case of ADPKD presenting initially with a solitary simple cyst.

Medullary Sponge Kidney

Medullary sponge kidney (MSK) is a nongenetically transmitted disease, characterized by ectasia of papillary collecting ducts in the renal medulla, congregating at the papillary tips, and involving

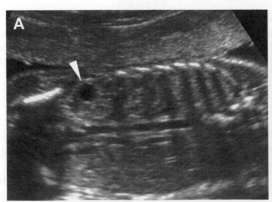
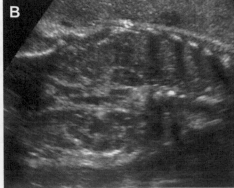

Fig. 61. Simple cyst with prenatal disappearance. (*A*) Routine obstetric US at 20 WGA shows a simple cyst in the left kidney (*arrowhead*). (*B*) Obstetric US at 32 WGA shows resolution of the left renal cyst. Postnatal renal US (not shown) was also normal.

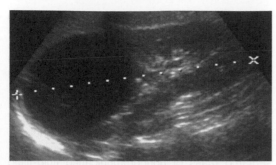

Fig. 62. Simple cyst;14-year-old girl with left flank pain. US shows a large cyst in the upper part of the left kidney. In situ sclerotherapy was performed.

one to all of pyramids. Papillary duct ectasia is for some a congenital (developmental) anomaly, discovered in adulthood when complications (renal lithiasis, urinary tract infection) have supervened, but for most is an acquired condition (because of its rarity in children). The liver is normal. Thirteen percent to 19% of adults with renal stones have underlying MSK. MSK is commonly detected in adults, whereas reported pediatric cases are rare. Kidneys are bilaterally (70% of cases) affected with normal size and intact function. Imaging (intravenous urography, CT, MR imaging) shows a characteristic radial linear streaking in the renal papillae. The ectatic or cystic papillary collecting ducts (spray-like pattern) have been compared with a "bouquet of flowers." The papillary streaking appearance is the key diagnostic criteria, detected in 0.5% to 2% of asymptomatic individuals undergoing renal imaging for assorted clinical conditions.

Sonography in pediatric cases of MSK has shown evidence of mild or moderate nephrocalcinosis[80,81] in kidneys of normal size, and a normal liver architecture (ie, different from ARPKD) (**Fig. 64**).

An association between MSK and hemihypertrophy has been emphasized: 25% of MSK patients have hemihypertrophy, 10% of patients with hemihypertrophy have MSK. Children with

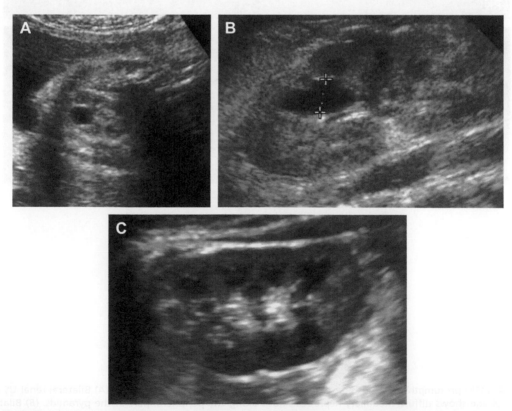

Fig. 63. Calyceal cyst versus simple cyst. (*A*) Obstetric US at 32 WGA shows a small cyst at the upper pole of the left kidney that remained unchanged from the 20 to 37 WGA sonograms. (*B*) Left renal US at 1 month of age shows the upper pole cystic lesion is adjacent to an upper pole calyx. (*C*) Follow-up US at 1 year of age shows a normal left kidney with cyst resolution.

MSK and hemihypertrophy may have an incomplete form of Beckwith-Wiedemann syndrome. Because of the increased risk of malignancies in patients with Beckwith-Wiedemann, or hemihypertrophy, these patients should be screened periodically by US for abdominal tumors.

Renal Cystic Neoplasms

Multilocular cystic renal tumor is a term that refers to two histologically distinct lesions that are indistinguishable preoperatively and perioperatively: cystic nephroma (CN) and cystic partially differentiated nephroblastoma (CPDN) (**Figs. 65–67**).[82–85]

CN (formerly "multilocular cystic nephroma") is a benign neoplasm encountered in children and in adults with a bimodal distribution of age and gender: 65% occur in patients less than 4 years of age with a male/female ratio of 2:1, 5% between 5 and 30 years of age, and 30% over 30 years of age with a female/male ratio of 8:1. Pathologic features are a solitary, well-circumscribed, multiseptated mass of noncommunicating fluid-filled locules with intercystic thin septa compressing the renal parenchyma.

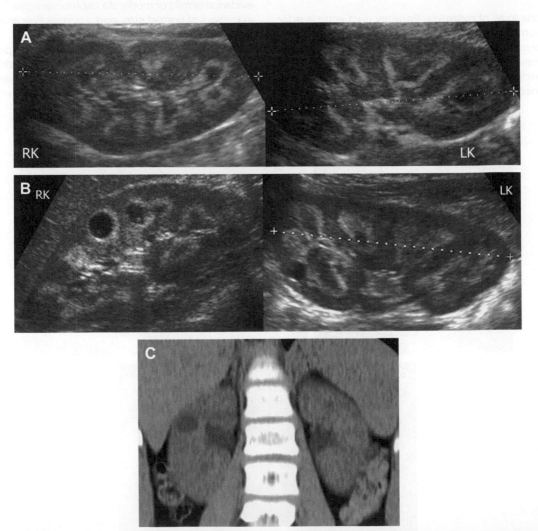

Fig. 64. MSK; presumptive diagnosis, as parents refused any contrast imaging study. (*A*) Bilateral renal US at 4 years of age shows diffuse medullary nephrocalcinosis along the peripheral part of the pyramids. (*B*) Bilateral renal US at 7 years of age shows an unchanged appearance, except for the appearance of two medullary cysts in the right kidney, and a cortical cyst in the left kidney. (*C*) Unenhanced renal CT showing the renal cysts. No calcium was apparent on CT. The liver was normal. Some cases of ADPKD coexisting with MSK have been reported in the literature.

CPDN has the same macroscopic appearance as CN and the same imaging features: at sonography, CN and CPDN present both as a multiloculated mass with thin septa and no solid elements. The septa enhance on postcontrast CT, without evidence of solid nodules.

CN and CPDN are treated by nephrectomy.[86] In CN, the septa do not contain blastemal cells, whereas CPDN shows the presence of septal blastema at histology. CPDN mostly affects boys and girls less than 2 years of age. CN and CPDN may be associated with pleuropulmonary blastoma.[87]

Four other neoplasms of childhood[88] may also appear as multilocular cystic masses: (1) Wilms tumor with cyst formation caused by hemorrhage and necrosis; (2) clear cell sarcoma (formerly called "anaplastic subtype of Wilms"); (3) cystic mesoblastic nephroma (cellular subtype)[89]; and

(4) cystic renal cell carcinoma. In most patients, nodular solid elements are also present at US and CT, in association with the cystic components (complex renal mass).

Intralobar nephrogenic rests sometimes exhibit cystic changes. Pathologically, cystic Wilms tumor, CPDN, and CN are considered to be intralobar nephrogenic rests–based lesions. Intralobar nephrogenic rests are associated with several conditions predisposing to the development of Wilms tumor (eg, aniridia, WAGR and Denys-Drash syndromes), whereas perilobar nephrogenic rests are usually found in Wilms associated with hemihypertrophy and Beckwith-Wiedemann syndrome. Nephroblastomatosis, the presence of multiple or diffuse nephrogenic rests,[90] may show cysts in association with solid nodules.

Finally, two nonneoplastic conditions may mimic a multicystic renal tumor in children: the

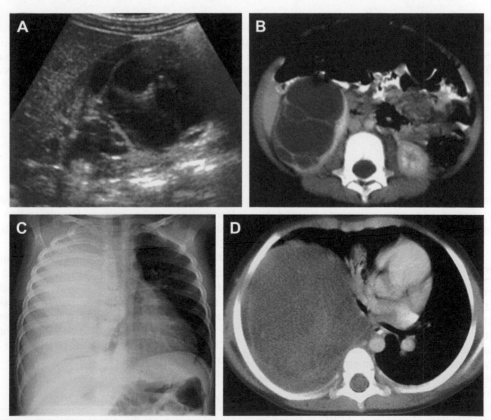

Fig. 65. CN; two year old presenting with simultaneous tumors in the right kidney and right lung (cystic nephroma and pleuropulmonary blastoma). (*A*) Longitudinal sonogram of the right kidney shows a lower pole multicystic mass. (*B*) Contrast-enhanced CT shows no solid components within the right renal cystic mass. (*C*) Chest radiograph shows complete opacification of the right hemithorax and mediastinal shift to the left. (*D*) Contrast-enhanced chest CT shows tumor filling the entire RT hemithorax.

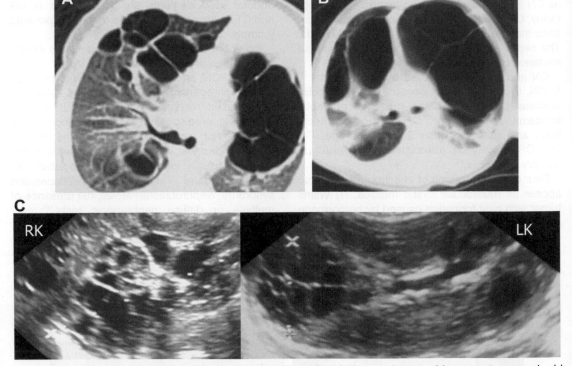

Fig. 66. Cystic partially differentiated nephroblastoma (CPDN) and pleuropulmonary blastoma. One-month-old boy referred for bilateral pulmonary cysts. Renal US was normal at presentation. (*A*) Chest CT at 1 month of age shows numerous thin-walled cysts. Surgical biopsy was not conclusive. (*B*) Follow-up chest CT at 5 months of age shows marked progression and enlargement of cysts. (*C*) Renal US at 5 months of age shows multiple, bilateral multicystic masses. Lung and renal biopsies confirmed bilateral pleuropulmonary blastoma and bilateral CPDN.

segmental multicystic dysplasia of a duplex kidney; and in very rare instances, a unilateral atypical presentation of ADPKD.

Acquired Cysts

Acquired cystic kidney disease (ACKD) is characterized by bilateral cystic changes distributed throughout the renal cortex and the medulla in patients with end-stage renal disease unrelated to inherited renal cystic diseases (**Figs. 68 and 69**). Cysts are usually small in size. Kidney size is variable, usually reduced, but at times normal or even increased.[91,92]

The prevalence and severity of ACKD increase with the duration of azotemia. ACKD is found in 7% to 22% of patients with end-stage renal disease before dialysis, in 58% of patients with 2 to 4 years of dialysis, 75% with 4 to 8 years, and in 92% with dialysis longer than 8 years. The cysts can regress after successful renal transplantation. Hemorrhage and neoplastic transformation (renal cell carcinoma) are the main complication of ACKD.

ACKD is notably less prevalent in children with end-stage renal disease than in azotemic adult patients. Accordingly, renal cysts demonstrated in the pediatric age group before dialysis are much more likely to be related to the underlying condition (eg, NPH) than to ACKD. In children, ACKD has also been reported after liver transplantation.[93]

Renal Cysts of Nontubular Origin

Renal sinus cysts (hilus cyst within sinus lipomatosis; parapelvic cyst of lymphatic origin) are common in adults, rarely seen in children. Perirenal lymphangiomas are rare, and have been observed in TSC patients.[94] Subcapsular and

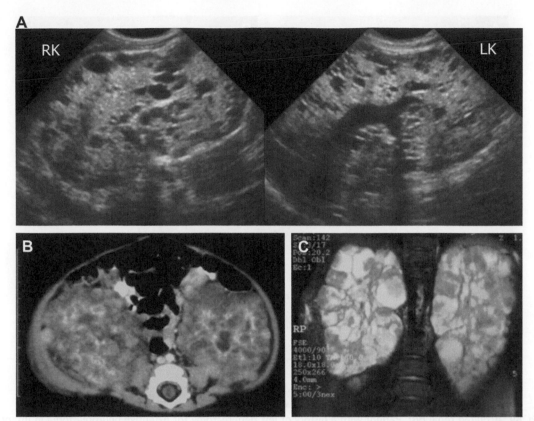

Fig. 67. Nephroblastomatosis. Three-month-old infant with bilateral renal masses. (*A*) Longitudinal sonograms of both kidneys shows multiple hypoechoic renal masses. (*B*) Contrast-enhanced CT shows enlarged kidneys with numerous areas of central and peripheral nonenhancement. (*C*) Coronal T2-weighted MRI shows diffuse involvement of both kidneys with complex solid and cystic masses. Surgical biopsy proved cystic nephroblastomatosis.

perirenal urinomas (uriniferous pseudocyst) are usually secondary to obstructive uropathies, either developmental (posterior urethral valves, ureteropelvic junction obstruction, ureterovesical junction obstruction) or acquired (ureteric calculus, trauma). Pyelocalyceal cysts and diverticula are probably developmental in origin, and subdivided into two types. Type I, more common, is connected to a minor calyx and located often in the poles (especially the upper). Type II represents a diverticulum from a major calyx or from the pelvis.

Pyelocalyceal cysts occur sporadically, affect all age groups, and usually are unilateral. At the time of intravenous urography, they were detected in 0.5% of cases. They only become symptomatic when complicated by nephrolithiasis, infection, or inflammation. In the latter instance, the cyst can enlarge markedly in relation to the obstruction

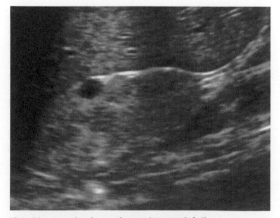

Fig. 68. Acquired renal cyst in renal failure. Ten year old with end-stage renal failure; renal transplantation was performed 2 years later. Longitudinal sonogram of the right kidney shows a small echogenic kidney with an acquired cortical cyst.

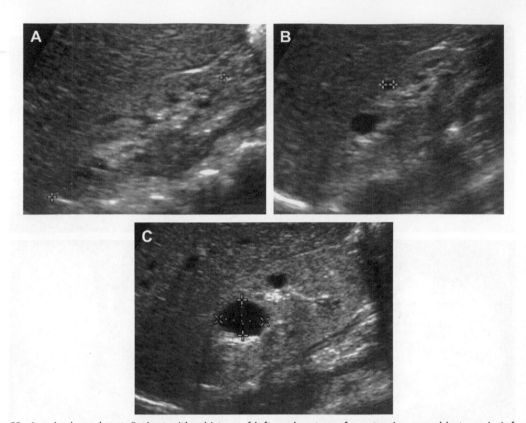

Fig. 69. Acquired renal cyst. Patient with a history of left nephrectomy for extensive neuroblastoma in infancy, and hemolytic uremic syndrome involving the remaining right kidney. (*A*) Longitudinal sonogram at 5 years of age shows a slightly echogenic right kidney measuring 7.1 cm. (*B*) Sonogram at 6 years of age show small acquired cysts. (*C*) Sonogram at 7 years of age shows enlarging cysts (*cursors*) and a renal length of 7.4 cm.

of the diverticulum's neck. The frequency of stone formation in calyceal diverticula is reported to be between 10% and 40%.

SUMMARY

Classification of cystic renal disease in children is based on the distinction between genetic and nongenetic disorders. US is the cornerstone of imaging in cystic renal disease.[95] The assessment of kidney size, laterality of involvement, parenchymal echogenicity, corticomedullary demarcation, cysts characteristics, and associated extrarenal abnormalities are often very contributive both at presentation (in utero or postnatally) and during follow-up. Suggestive sonographic patterns are seen especially in ARPKD, MCDK, various malformation syndromes, NPH, ORD, and multilocular cystic nephroma.

ACKNOWLEDGMENTS

I express my deep gratitude to Ginette Bleau for her support, kindness, and availability in formatting and editing the manuscript.

REFERENCES

1. Bisceglia M, Galliani CA, Senger C, et al. Renal cystic diseases: a review. Adv Anat Pathol 2006; 13(1):26–56.
2. Hartman DS. Renal cystic disease. In: Davidson AJ, editor. AFIP atlas of radiologic-pathologic correlation. Fascicule 1. Philadelphia: W.B. Saunders; 1989. p. 1–154.
3. Avner ED, Sweeney WE Jr. Renal cystic disease: new insights for the clinician. Pediatr Clin North Am 2006;53(5):889–909, ix.
4. Torres VE, Grantham JJ. Cystic diseases of the kidney. In: Brenner BM, Rector FC, editors. Brenner and rector's the kidney. 8th edition. Philadelphia: Saunders Elsevier; 2008. p. 1428–62.
5. Gagnadoux MF, Habib R, Levy M, et al. Cystic renal diseases in children. Adv Nephrol Necker Hosp 1989;18:33–57.
6. Zhang Q, Taulman PD, Yoder BK. Cystic kidney diseases: all roads lead to the cilium. Physiology (Bethesda) 2004;19:225–30.
7. Ong AC, Wheatley DN. Polycystic kidney disease: the ciliary connection. Lancet 2003;361(9359): 774–6.

8. Wang S, Luo Y, Wilson PD, et al. The autosomal recessive polycystic kidney disease protein is localized to primary cilia, with concentration in the basal body area. J Am Soc Nephrol 2004;15(3):592–602.

9. Pazour GJ. Intraflagellar transport and cilia-dependent renal disease: the ciliary hypothesis of polycystic kidney disease. J Am Soc Nephrol 2004; 15(10):2528–36.

10. Fliegauf M, Benzing T, Omran H. When cilia go bad: cilia defects and ciliopathies. Nat Rev Mol Cell Biol 2007;8(11):880–93.

11. Guay-Woodford LM. Renal cystic diseases: diverse phenotypes converge on the cilium/centrosome complex. Pediatr Nephrol 2006;21(10):1369–76.

12. de Bruyn R, Gordon I. Imaging in cystic renal disease. Arch Dis Child 2000;83(5):401–7.

13. Chakraborty S, McHugh K. Cystic diseases of the kidney in children. Imaging 2005;17:69–75.

14. Avni FE, Garel L, Cassart M, et al. Perinatal assessment of hereditary cystic renal diseases: the contribution of sonography. Pediatr Radiol 2006;36(5): 405–14.

15. Fick-Brosnahan G, Johnson AM, Strain JD, et al. Renal asymmetry in children with autosomal dominant polycystic kidney disease. Am J Kidney Dis 1999;34(4):639–45.

16. Bae KT, Zhu F, Chapman AB, et al. Magnetic resonance imaging evaluation of hepatic cysts in early autosomal-dominant polycystic kidney disease: the Consortium for Radiologic Imaging Studies of Polycystic Kidney Disease cohort. Clin J Am Soc Nephrol 2006;1(1):64–9.

17. Tee JB, Acott PD, McLellan DH, et al. Phenotypic heterogeneity in pediatric autosomal dominant polycystic kidney disease at first presentation: a single-center, 20-year review. Am J Kidney Dis 2004; 43(2):296–303.

18. Fick-Brosnahan GM, Tran ZV, Johnson AM, et al. Progression of autosomal-dominant polycystic kidney disease in children. Kidney Int 2001;59(5): 1654–62.

19. Grantham JJ, Torres VE, Chapman AB, et al. Volume progression in polycystic kidney disease. N Engl J Med 2006;354(20):2122–30.

20. Chapman AB, Guay-Woodford LM, Grantham JJ, et al. Renal structure in early autosomal-dominant polycystic kidney disease (ADPKD): the Consortium for Radiologic Imaging Studies of Polycystic Kidney Disease (CRISP) cohort. Kidney Int 2003;64(3): 1035–45.

21. Chapman AB. Autosomal dominant polycystic kidney disease: time for a change? J Am Soc Nephrol 2007;18(5):1399–407.

22. Boyer O, Gagnadoux MF, Guest G, et al. Prognosis of autosomal dominant polycystic kidney disease diagnosed in utero or at birth. Pediatr Nephrol 2007;22(3):380–8.

23. Fencl F, Janda J, Bláhová K, et al. Genotype-phenotype correlation in children with autosomal dominant polycystic kidney disease. Pediatr Nephrol 2009; 24(5):983–9.

24. Shamshirsaz AA, Reza Bekheirnia M, Kamgar M, et al. Autosomal-dominant polycystic kidney disease in infancy and childhood: progression and outcome. Kidney Int 2005;68(5):2218–24.

25. Strand WR, Rushton HG, Markle BM, et al. Autosomal dominant polycystic kidney disease in infants: asymmetric disease mimicking a unilateral renal mass. J Urol 1989;141(5):1151–3.

26. Shiroyanagi Y, Suzuki M, Matsuno D, et al. Asymmetric development of tumor-like cysts in a child with autosomal dominant polycystic kidney disease. J Pediatr Surg 2008;43(11):e21–3.

27. Brook-Carter PT, Peral B, Ward CJ, et al. Deletion of the TSC2 and PKD1 genes associated with severe infantile polycystic kidney disease: a contiguous gene syndrome. Nat Genet 1994;8(4):328–32.

28. Bisceglia M, Galliani C, Carosi I, et al. Tuberous sclerosis complex with polycystic kidney disease of the adult type: the TSC2/ADPKD1 contiguous gene syndrome. Int J Surg Pathol 2008;16(4): 375–85.

29. Brun M, Maugey-Laulom B, Eurin D, et al. Prenatal sonographic patterns in autosomal dominant polycystic kidney disease: a multicenter study. Ultrasound Obstet Gynecol 2004;24(1):55–61.

30. Ravine D, Gibson RN, Walker RG, et al. Evaluation of ultrasonographic diagnostic criteria for autosomal dominant polycystic kidney disease 1. Lancet 1994;343(8901):824–7.

31. Nicolau C, Torra R, Bianchi L, et al. Abdominal sonographic study of autosomal dominant polycystic kidney disease. J Clin Ultrasound 2000;28(6):277–82.

32. Guay-Woodford LM, Desmond RA. Autosomal recessive polycystic kidney disease: the clinical experience in North America. Pediatrics 2003; 111(5 Pt 1):1072–80.

33. Gunay-Aygun M, Avner ED, Bacallao RL, et al. Autosomal recessive polycystic kidney disease and congenital hepatic fibrosis: summary statement of a first National Institutes of Health/Office of Rare Diseases conference. J Pediatr 2006; 149(2):159–64.

34. Zerres K, Senderek J, Rudnik-Schöneborn S, et al. New options for prenatal diagnosis in autosomal recessive polycystic kidney disease by mutation analysis of the PKHD1 gene. Clin Genet 2004; 66(1):53–7.

35. Davis ID, Ho M, Hupertz V, et al. Survival of childhood polycystic kidney disease following renal transplantation: the impact of advanced hepatobiliary disease. Pediatr Transplant 2003;7(5):364–9.

36. Currarino G, Stannard MW, Rutledge JC. The sonolucent cortical rim in infantile polycystic kidneys:

histologic correlation. J Ultrasound Med 1989;8(10): 571–4.

37. Blickman JG, Bramson RT, Herrin JT. Autosomal recessive polycystic kidney disease: long-term sonographic findings in patients surviving the neonatal period. AJR Am J Roentgenol 1995; 164(5):1247–50.

38. Turkbey B, Ocak I, Daryanani K, et al. Autosomal recessive polycystic kidney disease and congenital hepatic fibrosis (ARPKD/CHF). Pediatr Radiol 2009; 39(2):100–11.

39. Lonergan GJ, Rice RR, Suarez ES. Autosomal recessive polycystic kidney disease: radiologic-pathologic correlation. Radiographics 2000;20(3): 837–55.

40. Avni FE, Guissard G, Hall M, et al. Hereditary polycystic kidney diseases in children: changing sonographic patterns through childhood. Pediatr Radiol 2002;32(3):169–74.

41. Traubici J, Daneman A. High-resolution renal sonography in children with autosomal recessive polycystic kidney disease. AJR Am J Roentgenol 2005; 184(5):1630–3.

42. Salomon R, Saunier S, Niaudet P. Nephronophthisis. Pediatr Nephrol 2009;24(12):2333–44.

43. Garel LA, Habib R, Pariente D, et al. Juvenile nephronophthisis: sonographic appearance in children with severe uremia. Radiology 1984;151(1):93–5.

44. Aguilera A, Rivera M, Gallego N, et al. Sonographic appearance of the juvenile nephronophthisis-cystic renal medulla complex. Nephrol Dial Transplant 1997;12(3):625–6.

45. Blowey DL, Querfeld U, Geary D, et al. Ultrasound findings in juvenile nephronophthisis. Pediatr Nephrol 1996;10(1):22–4.

46. Woolf AS, Feather SA, Bingham C. Recent insights into kidney diseases associated with glomerular cysts. Pediatr Nephrol 2002;17(4):229–35.

47. Bernstein J. Glomerulocystic kidney disease: nosological considerations. Pediatr Nephrol 1993;7(4): 464–70.

48. Sharp CK, Bergman SM, Stockwin JM, et al. Dominantly transmitted glomerulocystic kidney disease: a distinct genetic entity. J Am Soc Nephrol 1997; 8(1):77–84.

49. Cassart M, Eurin D, Didier F, et al. Antenatal renal sonographic anomalies and postnatal follow-up of renal involvement in Bardet-Biedl syndrome. Ultrasound Obstet Gynecol 2004;24(1):51–4.

50. Ickowicz V, Eurin D, Maugey-Laulom B, et al. Meckel-Grüber syndrome: sonography and pathology. Ultrasound Obstet Gynecol 2006;27(3):296–300.

51. Harker CP, Winter T III, Mack L. Prenatal diagnosis of Beckwith-Wiedemann syndrome. AJR Am J Roentgenol 1997;168(2):520–2.

52. Lonser RR, Glenn GM, Walther M, et al. von Hippel-Lindau disease. Lancet 2003;361(9374):2059–67.

53. Green JS, Parfrey PS, Harnett JD, et al. The cardinal manifestations of Bardet-Biedl syndrome, a form of Laurence-Moon-Biedl syndrome. N Engl J Med 1989;321(15):1002–9.

54. Thauvin-Robinet C, Cossée M, Cormier-Daire V, et al. Clinical, molecular, and genotype-phenotype correlation studies from 25 cases of oral-facial-digital syndrome type 1: a French and Belgian collaborative study. J Med Genet 2006;43(1):54–61.

55. Casper KA, Donnelly LF, Chen B, et al. Tuberous sclerosis complex: renal imaging findings. Radiology 2002;225(2):451–6.

56. Sampson JR, Maheshwar MM, Aspinwall R, et al. Renal cystic disease in tuberous sclerosis: role of the polycystic kidney disease 1 gene. Am J Hum Genet 1997;61(4):843–51.

57. Lendvay TS, Marshall FF. The tuberous sclerosis complex and its highly variable manifestations. J Urol 2003;169(5):1635–42.

58. O'Callaghan FJ, Noakes MJ, Martyn CN, et al. An epidemiological study of renal pathology in tuberous sclerosis complex. BJU Int 2004;94(6):853–7.

59. Salame H, Damry N, Vandenhoudt K, et al. The contribution of ultrasound for the differential diagnosis of congenital and infantile nephrotic syndrome. Eur Radiol 2003;13(12):2674–9.

60. Winyard P, Chitty LS. Dysplastic kidneys. Semin Fetal Neonatal Med 2008;13(3):142–51.

61. Matsell DG. Renal dysplasia: new approaches to an old problem. Am J Kidney Dis 1998;32(4): 535–43.

62. Haecker FM, Wehrmann M, Hacker HW, et al. Renal dysplasia in children with posterior urethral valves: a primary or secondary malformation? Pediatr Surg Int 2002;18(2–3):119–22.

63. Decramer S, Parant O, Beaufils S, et al. Anomalies of the TCF2 gene are the main cause of fetal bilateral hyperechogenic kidneys. J Am Soc Nephrol 2007; 18(3):923–33.

64. Weber S, Moriniere V, Knüppel T, et al. Prevalence of mutations in renal developmental genes in children with renal hypodysplasia: results of the ESCAPE study. J Am Soc Nephrol 2006;17(10):2864–70.

65. Zaffanello M, Brugnara M, Franchini M, et al. TCF2 gene mutation leads to nephro-urological defects of unequal severity: an open question. Med Sci Monit 2008;14(6):RA78–86.

66. Oliveira EA, Diniz JS, Vilasboas AS, et al. Multicystic dysplastic kidney detected by fetal sonography: conservative management and follow-up. Pediatr Surg Int 2001;17(1):54–7.

67. Eckoldt F, Woderich R, Smith RD, et al. Antenatal diagnostic aspects of unilateral multicystic kidney dysplasia: sensitivity, specificity, predictive values, differential diagnoses, associated malformations and consequences. Fetal Diagn Ther 2004;19(2): 163–9.

68. Woolf AS. Unilateral multicystic dysplastic kidney. Kidney Int 2006;69(1):190–3.

69. Welch TR, Wacksman J. The changing approach to multicystic dysplastic kidney in children. J Pediatr 2005;146(6):723–5.

70. Kalyoussef E, Hwang J, Prasad V, et al. Segmental multicystic dysplastic kidney in children. Urology 2006;68(5):1121: e9–11.

71. Rabelo EA, Oliveira EA, Diniz JS, et al. Natural history of multicystic kidney conservatively managed: a prospective study. Pediatr Nephrol 2004;19(10):1102–7.

72. Aslam M, Watson AR. Trent and Anglia MCDK Study Group. Unilateral multicystic dysplastic kidney: long term outcomes. Arch Dis Child 2006;91(10):820–3.

73. Rottenberg GT, Gordon I, De Bruyn R. The natural history of the multicystic dysplastic kidney in children. Br J Radiol 1997;70(832):347–50.

74. Strife JL, Souza AS, Kirks DR, et al. Multicystic dysplastic kidney in children: US follow-up. Radiology 1993;186(3):785–8.

75. Onal B, Kogan BA. Natural history of patients with multicystic dysplastic kidney: what followup is needed? J Urol 2006;176(4 Pt 1):1607–11.

76. Chaumoitre K, Brun M, Cassart M, et al. Differential diagnosis of fetal hyperechogenic cystic kidneys unrelated to renal tract anomalies: a multicenter study. Ultrasound Obstet Gynecol 2006;28(7):911–7.

77. Terada N, Ichioka K, Matsuta Y, et al. The natural history of simple renal cysts. J Urol 2002;167(1):21–3.

78. McHugh K, Stringer DA, Hebert D, et al. Simple renal cysts in children: diagnosis and follow-up with US. Radiology 1991;178(2):383–5.

79. Blazer S, Zimmer EZ, Blumenfeld Z, et al. Natural history of fetal simple renal cysts detected in early pregnancy. J Urol 1999;162(3 Pt 1):812–4.

80. Patriquin HB, O'Regan S. Medullary sponge kidney in childhood. AJR Am J Roentgenol 1985;145(2):315–9.

81. Talenti E, Lubrano G, Pavanello L, et al. Medullary sponge kidney in childhood: the diagnostic contribution of echography. Radiol Med 1989;77(3):290–2.

82. Joshi VV, Beckwith JB. Multilocular cyst of the kidney (cystic nephroma) and cystic, partially differentiated nephroblastom: terminology and criteria for diagnosis. Cancer 1989;64(2):466–79.

83. Agrons GA, Wagner BJ, Davidson AJ, et al. Multilocular cystic renal tumor in children: radiologic-pathologic correlation. Radiographics 1995;15(3):653–69.

84. van den Hoek J, de Krijger R, van de Ven K, et al. Cystic nephroma, cystic partially differentiated nephroblastoma and cystic Wilms' tumor in children: a spectrum with therapeutic dilemmas. Urol Int 2009;82(1):65–70.

85. Boybeyi O, Karnak I, Orhan D, et al. Cystic nephroma and localized renal cystic disease in children: diagnostic clues and management. J Pediatr Surg 2008;43(11):1985–9.

86. Blakely ML, Shamberger RC, Norkool P, et al. Outcome of children with cystic partially differentiated nephroblastoma treated with or without chemotherapy. Pediatr Surg 2003;38(6):897–900.

87. Boman F, Hill DA, Williams GM, et al. Familial association of pleuropulmonary blastoma with cystic nephroma and other renal tumors: a report from the International Pleuropulmonary Blastoma Registry. J Pediatr 2006;149:850–4.

88. Argani P, Ladanyi M. Recent advances in pediatric renal neoplasia. Adv Anat Pathol 2003;10(5):243–60.

89. Drut R. Multicystic congenital mesoblastic nephroma. Int J Surg Pathol 2002;10(1):59–63.

90. Hennigar RA, O'Shea PA, Grattan-Smith JD. Clinicopathologic features of nephrogenic rests and nephroblastomatosis. Adv Anat Pathol 2001;8(5):276–89.

91. Levine E. Acquired cystic kidney disease. Radiol Clin North Am 1996;34(5):947–64.

92. Choyke PL. Acquired cystic kidney disease. Eur Radiol 2000;10(11):1716–21.

93. Calvo-Garcia MA, Campbell KM, O'Hara SM, et al. Acquired renal cysts after pediatric liver transplantation: association with cyclosporine and renal dysfunction. Pediatr Transplant 2008;12(6):666–71.

94. Torres VE, Björnsson J, King BF, et al. Extrapulmonary lymphangioleiomyomatosis and lymphangiomatous cysts in tuberous sclerosis complex. Mayo Clin Proc 1995;70(7):641–8.

95. Vester U, Kranz B, Hoyer PF. The diagnostic value of ultrasound in cystic kidney diseases. Pediatr Nephrol 2008. [Epub ahead of print].

Scrotal Ultrasound

Boaz Karmazyn, MD

KEYWORDS

- Ultrasound • Pediatric • Scrotum • Testis
- Acute scrotum • Scrotal mass

Ultrasound (US) is a readily available and relatively inexpensive imaging modality that can be performed on patients at any age without the need for sedation or any other pretest preparation.[1–4] US examinations are safe and there is no significant biologic risk from radiation exposure.[1–4] Gray-scale US provides high-resolution depiction of scrotal anatomy and Doppler technique demonstrates perfusion.[1–4]

Different pathologies of the scrotum may have similar clinical presentation, such as acute scrotal pain or scrotal mass. US of the scrotum can better guide treatment by improving the definition of the scrotal pathology.[1–4] For these reasons, US became the imaging modality of choice for evaluation of scrotal pathology, and, in most cases, US is the first and only imaging needed for evaluation of scrotal pathology.[1–4]

ANATOMY

The scrotum is divided by the midline raphe. Each half of the scrotum contains a spermatic cord, testis, and epididymis. The testes descend into the scrotum at approximately the 28th gestational week via the inguinal canal through the peritoneal recess, which is called the processus vaginalis. The processus vaginalis gradually closes through infancy and childhood. The testis is covered by a visceral layer of tunica vaginalis, except where in contact with epididymis, and by the tunica albuginea. The posterior surface of the tunica albuginea extends into the testis to form the mediastinum testis. This is seen as a middle echogenic line on longitudinal US of the testis (**Fig. 1**). The testis has lobules containing the seminiferous tubules. Testicular lobules are occasionally identified as lines radiating from the mediastinum testis (**Fig. 2**).[1,4]

The size and shape of the testes change with age. Testicular size is influenced by gonadal hormones. In boys, from birth to 5 months of age, the testicular volume rises to a maximum of 0.44 ($\pm$0.03) cm^3.[5] The rise in testicular volume coincides with a peak in gonadotropic hormones, so-called minipuberty, at approximately 3 to 4 months of age.[6,7] After age 5 months, the testicular volume steadily declines and reaches its minimum volume at approximately 9 months of age and remains approximately the same size until puberty.[5] The testis is rounded in newborns and gradually becomes ovoid with growth.[5] The echogenicity of the testis increases in puberty due to the development of germ cell elements.[1,2] US evaluation of testicular volume is more precise, especially in infants, compared with the orchidometer evaluation. The smallest bead in the Prader orchidometer is 1 cm^3, whereas the US-measured volumes in the first years of life are typically less than 0.5 cm^3. In addition, the orchidometer overestimates testicular volume as it measures not only the testis but also the epididymis and the hydrocele (if present) and the scrotal skin.[8]

Color Doppler demonstrates capsular and intratesticular vessels. In prepubertal testes, it can be difficult to detect intratesticular flow, but the capsular arteries are easier to identify. It is, however, the author's experience that with the use of state-of-the-art US equipment and settings, intratesticular flow can be detected in almost all testes at any patient age. The resistive index of the intratesticular arteries changes with age from high to low resistive index (**Fig. 3**).[1,2]

The epididymis has three parts: head, body, and tail. In the normal epididymis, only the head is routinely identified. The epididymal head is located in the upper pole of the scrotum, is triangular in shape, and has the same echogenicity as the testis (see **Fig. 1**).[1,4]

Department of Pediatric Radiology, Riley Hospital for Children, Indiana University School of Medicine, 702 Barnhill Drive, Room 1053, Indianapolis, IN 46202, USA
E-mail address: bkarmazy@iupui.edu

Ultrasound Clin 5 (2010) 61–74
doi:10.1016/j.cult.2009.11.009
1556-858X/10/$ – see front matter © 2010 Elsevier Inc. All rights reserved.

ultrasound.theclinics.com

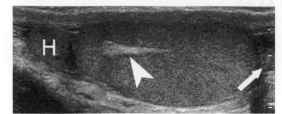

Fig. 1. Normal anatomy of the scrotum. Longitudinal scan of a normal testis in a 17-year-old boy demonstrates homogeneous echo-texture with an echogenic mediastinum testis (*arrowhead*), epididymal head (H), and tail (*arrow*).

Testicular appendixes are remnants of the mesonephric and paramesonephric ducts. They can be identified by US in cases of hydrocele (**Fig. 4**).[1,4]

The spermatic cord appears as an echogenic band on longitudinal images and ovoid on transverse images as it passes in the inguinal canal. Color Doppler shows the testicular artery and pampiniform venous plexus (**Fig. 5**). In the inguinal canal, the normal thickness of the spermatic cord is up to 4 mm.[9] The normal inguinal canal does not contain fluid.

ULTRASOUND TECHNIQUE

The child lies on his back on the examination table. The penis is lifted up onto the abdomen and covered. In infancy and early childhood, when the processus vaginalis is open, it is useful to apply gentle pressure with a fingertip just above the scrotum in the inguinal canal to fixate the testis. In older boys, a rolled towel is placed between the legs to support the scrotum.

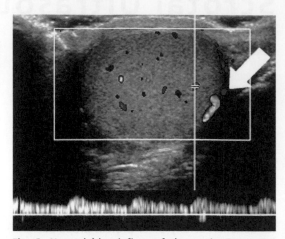

Fig. 3. Normal blood flow of the testis. Transverse duplex study demonstrates the normal capsular vessels (*arrow*) and normal testicular vessels with low-resistance arterial waveforms.

A linear transducer should be used and multiple longitudinal and transverse images of the testis should be performed. The gel should be warm. Testicular echotexture and shape should be evaluated. Testicular echotexture should be optimally compared in a dual view that demonstrates both testicles in the same view. Testicular volume should be measured using the volume = $L \times W \times H \times 0.52$, where L is testicular length, W is width, and H is height. Epididymal head, presence of hydrocele, and scrotal wall should be documented. Evaluation of varicocele or reducible hernia should be performed with and without Valsalva maneuver

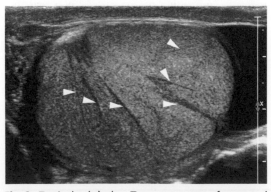

Fig. 2. Testicular lobules. Transverse scan of a normal testis in a 17-year-old boy demonstrates hypoechogenic lines (*arrowheads*) radiating from the mediastinum testis representing testicular lobule septations.

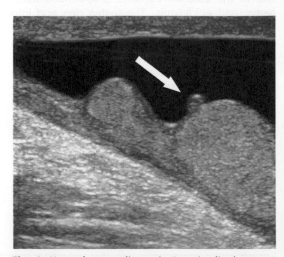

Fig. 4. Normal appendix testis. Longitudinal scan at the upper pole of the scrotum in a 2-month-old boy evaluated for hydrocele demonstrates a nodule (*arrow*) in the upper pole of the testis compatible with testicular appendix.

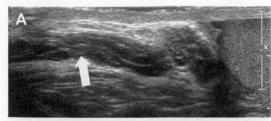

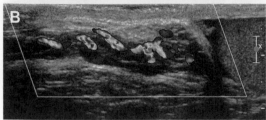

Fig. 5. Normal anatomy of the inguinal canal. Longitudinal scans demonstrate (*A*) the hypoechoic spermatic cord (*arrow*) and (*B*) the pampiniform venous plexus.

(children can be asked to blow a balloon). Additional images in the upright position may also be performed. Routine US of the scrotum should include evaluation of the inguinal canal.[1–4]

Color Doppler US should be performed with low wall filtration, low velocity scale, and by maximizing the color gain just below the level at which artifacts appear. The color region of interest size should be tailored to the size of the testis. Power Doppler should be used if no flow is identified by color Doppler US. Flow within the testicular vessels should be confirmed with spectral Doppler. Arterial and venous flow should be demonstrated. Maximal arterial velocity can be evaluated using angle correction.[1–4] Seldom, when it is difficult to trace intratesticular vascular flow in small boys, a cine-loop of the color Doppler study can help to differentiate between artifacts and true flow.

THE ACUTE SCROTUM

Acute scrotal pain is a medical urgency as 12% to 26% of boys who have it have testicular torsion.[10,11] The main differential diagnosis includes testicular torsion, torsion of appendix testis, and epididymitis. It is crucial to rapidly diagnose testicular torsion because prognosis of the testis depends on the duration of torsion.[12] Ischemia of the testis can be reversible in the first 6 hours.[12] US is typically required when the clinical assessment is equivocal for testicular torsion.

Testicular Torsion

Based on anatomy and age, testicular torsion is divided into intravaginal and extravaginal torsion. Intravaginal torsion is the most common type of torsion and occurs in older boys with a peak at approximately age 13.[12]

The underlying cause of intravaginal torsion is termed *bell clapper deformity* because the testis hangs freely within the tunica vaginalis. This is secondary to failure of posterior attachment to the tunica vaginalis.[1–4] When torsion occurs, the spermatic cord twists within the tunica vaginalis. The anatomic abnormality is bilateral in nearly 80% of the patients.[12]

Testicular torsion typically presents as an acute, excruciating scrotal pain of short duration before a patient arrives in the emergency room. Physical examination typically reveals diffuse tenderness, abnormal high and horizontal position of the testis, and absence of the cremasteric reflex.[1–4,10–12]

When clinical presentation and physical examination findings highly suggest the diagnosis of testicular torsion, scrotal exploration should be promptly performed. In many cases, however, symptoms and findings on physical examination are equivocal. In these cases, US provides a rapid, noninvasive evaluation of acute scrotal pain.[13]

Gray-scale findings of testicular torsion may be normal. Testicular gray-scale abnormalities include testicular swelling or heterogeneous or decreased testicular echotexture.[1–4] Heterogeneous parenchymal echotexture usually indicates testicular nonviability.[14] Other findings include swelling of the epididymis, hydrocele, and scrotal skin edema (**Fig. 6**).[1–4,13,15] Epididymal swelling is common in testicular torsion and, in a few cases,

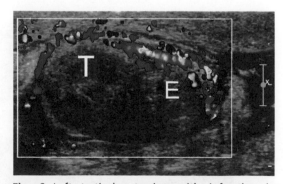

Fig. 6. Left testicular torsion with infarction in a 5-year-old boy. Longitudinal color Doppler scan demonstrates a swollen heterogeneous testis (T) and swollen epididymis (E). There is increased capsular vascularity but no intratesticular blood flow. This testis was not salvageable.

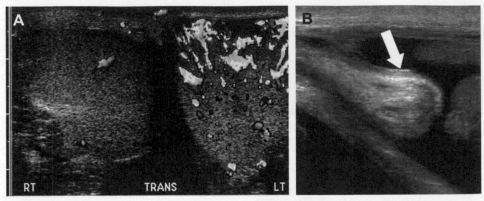

Fig. 7. Right testicular torsion in a 14-year-old boy. (*A*) Transverse color Doppler scan demonstrates markedly decreased right testicular flow. (*B*) Longitudinal scan in the upper pole of the right scrotum demonstrates thickening of the spermatic cord (*arrow*) with alternating hypo- and hyperechoic layers compatible with spermatic cord torsion. On scrotal exploration, there was 90° of spermatic cord torsion.

associated with increased epididymal flow. This should not mislead to the diagnosis of epididymitis.[13,15]

A gray-scale study should include evaluation of the spermatic cord (**Fig. 7**). A coiled spermatic cord could be the only sign for testicular torsion as perfusion of the testis can be normal in partial torsion (<360°) or even increased in a case of torsion-detorsion. Evaluation of the spermatic cord increases the sensitivity for detection of testicular torsion.[13,16–18]

Decreased testicular blood flow on a color Doppler study is the most sensitive finding that indicates testicular torsion.[1–4] Testicular capsular blood flow may increase and erroneously suggest, in young boys, the presence of testicular perfusion. Therefore, prudent examination of intratesticular blood flow is necessary. Spectral evaluation of the blood flow and documentation

of venous and arterial wave flow are important. Initially, only venous flow may be absent. Comparing the intratesticular flow to the contralateral testis is important, as any decrease in perfusion or change in the waveform may be the first indication of testicular torsion (see **Fig. 7**).[1–4,13]

Some investigators advocate US-guided manual detorsion of the testis to decrease the time of testicular ischemia.[19] Most commonly, the spermatic cord torsion is medial; therefore, the first attempt for manual detorsion should be performed by twisting the testis to the lateral side.[20] Surgery includes scrotal exploration, detorsion, and orchipexy of both testes.

Testicular torsion in the perinatal period, before or shortly after birth, is rare. This condition is due to loose attachments of the tunica to the scrotal wall; therefore, the torsion is called extratesticular. Perinatal testicular torsion appears as asymptomatic

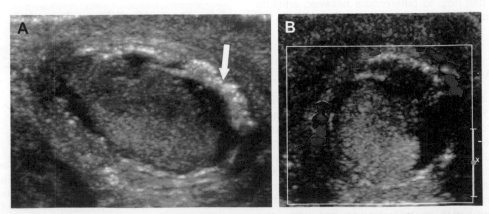

Fig. 8. Swollen testis secondary to perinatal testicular torsion. (*A*) Longitudinal scan demonstrates a swollen scrotal wall, calcification of the tunica vaginalis (*arrow*), and a swollen heterogeneous testis. (*B*) Transverse color Doppler demonstrates increased peritesticular flow but no intratesticular vascularity.

swelling of the scrotum with scrotal edema and discoloration. The testis is usually nonsalvageable. US findings depend on the stage of the torsion. Initially, the testis appears enlarged and heterogeneous (**Fig. 8**). In the chronic phase, the testis may have a peripheral rim of calcification and may be atrophic (**Fig. 9**).[21]

Torsion of Testicular Appendix

The appendix testis, a müllerian duct remnant located at the superior pole of the testicle, is the most common appendix to twist. The epididymal appendix, located at the head of the epididymis, is a wolffian duct remnant.[1–4]

Torsion of testicular appendix can occur at any age but is most common between the ages of 7 and 12 years. The pain is typically indolent and not as severe as the pain from testicular torsion. Duration of scrotal pain is significantly longer than that of testicular torsion. A palpable tender nodule in the upper pole of the scrotum and the blue dot sign, which represents the bluish discoloration of the torsed appendix, are specific signs for torsion of testicular appendix. In most boys, however, physical examination does not detect these signs.[1–4,22]

US typically demonstrates an extratesticular nodule with no vascularity in the upper pole of the scrotum. The nodule echotexture varies, but it is most commonly hyperechogenic (**Fig. 10**). The maximal diameter of the torsed appendix varies from 4 to 16 mm. There may be an overlap between the size of torsed and normal appendixes when the nodule is smaller than 6 mm.[22]

The torsed appendix leads to secondary inflammation in the surrounding structures. The epididymis is almost always swollen with increased perfusion, and occasionally there is swelling and

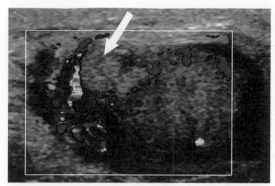

Fig. 10. Torsion of appendix testis in a 9-year-old boy. Longitudinal color Doppler scan demonstrates an echogenic extratesticular nodule with no vascularity (*arrow*) representing a torsed appendix testis with a reactive swollen epididymis with increased vascularity and scrotal wall edema.

increased perfusion of the testis. Other findings include scrotal wall edema and hydrocele. In some cases, when the torsed appendix is not identified by US, the findings cannot be distinguished from acute epididymitis.[23]

Treatment includes analgesic and anti-inflammatory medications. Surgery is reserved for patients in excruciating pain who are not responding to medication or when it is not possible to clinically distinguish from testicular torsion.

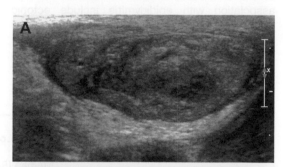

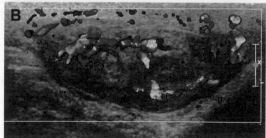

Fig. 11. Recurrent epididymitis in an 8-year-old boy who had two-stage hypospadias repair complicated by urethrocutaneous fistula and meatal stenosis. (*A*) Longitudinal gray-scale and (*B*) color Doppler scans demonstrate marked epididymal swelling and heterogeneity associated with increased vascularity.

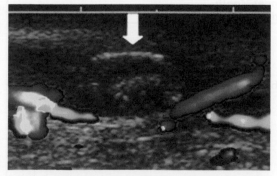

Fig. 9. Atrophic testis secondary to perinatal testicular torsion. Longitudinal scan demonstrates an atrophic testis and capsular calcifications (*arrow*) with no intratesticular blood flow.

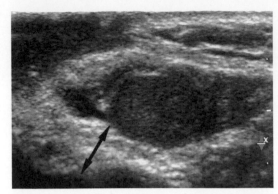

Fig. 12. Idiopathic scrotal edema in a 6-year-old boy. Transverse scan demonstrates a normal left testis with marked scrotal wall edema (*double arrowheads*). Similar findings were seen on the right side.

Acute Epididymitis

Epididymitis is an inflammation of the epididymis. Epididymitis is described in response to infection, trauma, vasculitis, or urine refluxing into the ejaculatory ducts but in most cases is idiopathic.[24] The diagnosis is often based on clinical presentation of a few days of acute scrotal pain, swelling, and tenderness of the epididymis.[24]

Presentation in young boys and those with recurrent epididymitis should lead to further evaluation with renal US and cystourethrography for associated anomalies. Anomalies that are described in association with epididymitis include ectopic ureter to the seminal vesicles and lower urinary tract anomalies, such as recto-ureteral fistula and strictures of the urethra. Recurrent epididymitis can also occur in boys with neurogenic bladder or functional bladder abnormalities.[24–28]

Gray-scale US findings of epididymo-orchitis include an enlarged epididymis. The echotexture of the epididymis varies, depending on time of evolution, from decreased to increased echogenicity. Inflammation of the testis, orchitis, is confirmed by enlarged testis with heterogeneous echotexture. Indirect signs of inflammation, such as reactive scrotal wall edema and hydrocele, are present in most cases. Duplex US demonstrates hyperemia of the epididymis and, when orchitis is present, increased testicular perfusion (**Fig. 11**).[1–4,28]

Acute Idiopathic Scrotal Edema

Acute idiopathic scrotal edema is an uncommon, self-limited disease of unknown origin. It is thought to be a variant of angioneurotic edema. It presents with unilateral or bilateral scrotal swelling without pain. Some boys have eosinophilia. Physical examination findings include skin swelling and erythema that involve the scrotum but can also extend to the inguinal and perianal area. Acute idiopathic scrotal edema is a diagnosis of exclusion.

US is helpful to confirm the diagnosis and prevent unnecessary scrotal exploration. Gray-scale US demonstrates marked scrotal skin edema with normal testis and epididymis. Color Doppler may show increased scrotal wall perfusion (**Fig. 12**).[29]

SCROTAL MASSES

Scrotal tumors are rare in boys and occur at an incidence of 0.5 to 2 per 100,000 boys.[30–32] Most boys with scrotal tumors present with a painless mass. On examination, the masses are typically firm. When a palpable mass is evaluated with

Table 1
Testicular tumors based on a summary of the prepubertal testis tumor registry

Tumor Type	Median (Range) Month at Presentation	Relative Frequency
Germ cell tumors		
Yolk sac	16 (0–131)	62%
Teratoma	13 (0–111)	23%
Epidermoid cyst	Not applicable	3%
Stromal tumors		
Juvenile granulosa	0.1 (0–6)	3%
Sertoli's cell	6 (4–121)	3%
Leydig's cell	66 (24–126)	1%
Unspecified stromal	4 (0–111)	4%
Gonadoblastoma	Not applicable	1%

Data from Ross JH, Rybicki L, Kay R. Clinical behavior and a contemporary management algorithm for prepubertal testis tumors: a summary of the Prepubertal Testis Tumor Registry. J Urol 2002;168(4 Pt 2):1675–8 [discussion: 1678–9].

US, the primary goal is localization of the mass (intratesticular or extratesticular) and further characterization of the mass.[1–4,33]

Intratesticular Tumors

Most of the intratesticular tumors present within the first 2 years and are germ cell tumors. According to the Prepubertal Testis Tumor Registry, the majority of the germ cell tumors are yolk sac, followed by teratoma (**Table 1**).[30] Stromal cell tumors are uncommon and can present with precocious puberty. Gonadoblastoma is a rare tumor that occurs in phenotypic females with 46,XY karyotype and intra-abdominal masses.[30–32]

Children with an intratesticular mass should be evaluated for signs of precocious puberty. Measurement of α-fetoprotein (AFP) should be performed as part of the initial evaluation. Most intratesticular tumors in the prepubertal testis are benign. Therefore, in some cases, testis-sparing surgery is an option. Except in boys with elevated AFP, evaluation for metastatic disease with chest radiograph and abdominal and pelvic CT is performed only after pathologic diagnosis of the malignant mass.[30–32]

Germ cell tumors

Germ cell tumors most commonly present within the first 2 years of life. A yolk sac tumor, also called an endodermal sinus tumor, accounts for 70% of prepubertal germ cell tumors. AFP is a reliable tumor marker that is increased in more than 80% of the cases. The serum levels of AFP should return to normal after 1 month after mass resection. Persistent elevation of AFP indicates metastatic disease and evaluation with chest radiographs and CT of the abdomen and pelvis should be performed. Metastases are usually hematogenous to the lungs. Lymphatic spread to the retroperitoneal

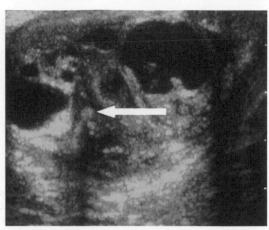

Fig. 14. Testicular teratoma in an infant. Longitudinal scan of the testis demonstrates a heterogeneous mass with solid and cystic components and a focus of calcification with shadowing (*arrow*).

lymph nodes is unusual and present in only 4% to 6% of cases. Retroperitoneal lymph node resection is performed in boys with elevated AFP and detection of enlarged retroperitoneal lymph nodes on the CT study.[30–32] Scrotal US demonstrates a solid testicular mass. In some cases, there is no definite mass but rather diffuse testicular enlargement (**Fig. 13**).[33]

Prepubertal teratomas are uniformly benign. Prepubertal boys can be treated with testis-sparing surgery. In adults, teratomas are considered malignant. Postpubertal boys should be treated as adults with complete orchiectomy. Typical US findings include heterogeneous mass with cystic component and calcifications (**Fig. 14**).[30–32,34]

An epidermoid cyst is a benign tumor of ectodermal origin composed of keratin-producing

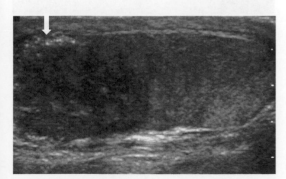

Fig. 13. Germ cell testicular tumor in a 15-year-old boy with hypospadias and cryptorchydism. Right scrotal longitudinal scan demonstrates hypoechoic mass in the upper pole of the testis associated with focal microlithiasis (*arrow*).

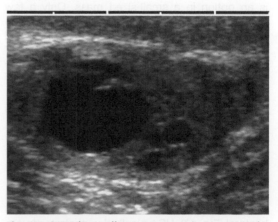

Fig. 15. Granulosa cell tumor presenting as testicular mass in a 4-month-old boy. Longitudinal scan demonstrates a complex solid and cystic mass.

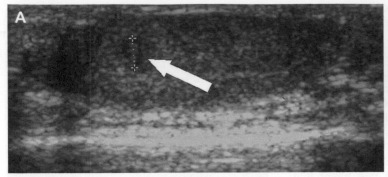
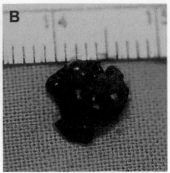

Fig. 16. Nonpalpable Leydig's cell tumor presenting as precocious puberty in an 8-year-old boy. (*A*) Longitudinal scan demonstrates a subtle 8-mm hypoechogenic focus (*arrow*) in the testis. (*B*) Surgical testicular preservation surgery was performed under US guidance with resection of the mass.

epithelium. US findings show typical characteristics and include a well-circumscribed, round cyst with layered echogenic debris. The treatment of choice is testis-sparing surgery. No follow-up US imaging is needed after surgery.[34,35]

Stromal cell tumors

Juvenile granulosa cell tumors are benign tumors that usually present in the first 6 months of life. They are associated with anomalies of the Y chromosome, mosaicism, and ambiguous genitalia. US typically demonstrates a multiseptated, hypoechoic mass (**Fig. 15**). Testis-sparing surgery is an option if there is an adequate amount of salvageable testicular parenchyma.[31,32,34]

Sertoli's cell tumors are rare. Some of the tumors secrete hormones that can present as gynecomastia or precocious puberty. All reported masses in boys younger than 5 years have been benign. Therefore, boys younger than 5 years can be treated with orchiectomy without imaging evaluation for metastasis. Testis-sparing surgery is an option in a small-sized mass. Only a few malignant Sertoli's tumors have been reported in boys older than 5 years. These boys should be evaluated with chest radiographs and CT scan of the abdomen and pelvis to evaluate for metastasis.[32]

Leydig's cell tumor is rare. It is benign in prepubertal boys. The tumor secretes 17-ketosteroids and these boys have high testosterone levels. Most present with precocious puberty and a few with gynecomastia. In prepubertal boys, treatment is with testis-sparing surgery or orchiectomy (**Fig. 16**).[31,32,34]

Leukemia and lymphoma are the most common metastatic tumors to the testis. They are often bilateral (**Fig. 17**). US typically demonstrates hypoechoic masses or uniform swelling of the testis with decreased echogenicity. At presentation,

testicular metastasis in acute lymphocytic leukemia usually signifies poor prognosis. After the central nervous system, the testis is the second most common extramedullary site of recurrence of leukemia. Treatment of relapsed leukemia includes local radiation and systemic chemotherapy.[31,32]

Gonadoblastoma

Gonadoblastomas are rare tumors discovered in phenotypic females with 46,XY karyotype and intra-abdominal testis. These tumors contain elements of germ cell and stromal cell tumors.

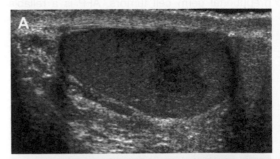

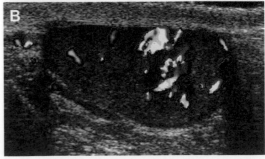

Fig. 17. Abdominal Burkitt's lymphoma with metastasis to the testes in a 13-year-old boy. (*A*) Longitudinal gray-scale and (*B*) color Doppler scans of the right testis demonstrate multifocal hypoechoic hypervascular testicular masses.

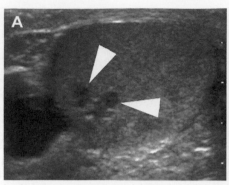 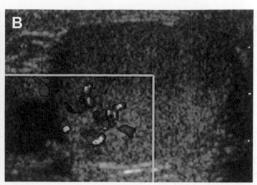

Fig. 18. A 12-year-old boy with congenital adrenal hyperplasia and bilateral adrenal rests. (*A*) Longitudinal scan of the right testis demonstrates peripheral hypoechoic nodules near the mediastinum testis (*arrowheads*). (*B*) Color Doppler scan demonstrates increased vascularity of the nodules.

These tumors are benign in newborns but may undergo malignant transformation to dysgerminoma during puberty.[31,32]

Due to the rare occurrence of gonadoblastomas and the value of the intra-abdominal testis in producing hormones, the current approach is periodic screening by imaging and physical examination rather than routine resection of the testes.

Other testicular benign lesions

There are various benign testicular masses that can mimic a testicular tumor.[36] These include adrenal rests in patients with increased adrenocortical hormones, mainly in congenital adrenal hyperplasia. On US, these lesions typically appear as bilateral multifocal hypoechoic nodules with increased vascularity (**Fig. 18**).[36,37] Other lesions include Leydig's cell hyperplasia, ectasia of the rete testis (**Fig. 19**), and intratesticular varicocele.[36]

Paratesticular Tumors

Paratesticular tumors usually arise from the connective tissue that supports the testis. Those can be benign tumors, such as leiomyoma, fibroma, lipoma, and hemangioma, or malignant tumors, such as leiomyosarcoma, fibrosarcoma, liposarcoma, and rhabdomyosarcoma. Except for rhabdomyosarcoma, these tumors are rare.[32]

Seventy-five percent of all rhabdomyosarcomas in boys are paratesticular (**Fig. 20**). They usually present with a painless scrotal mass and have bimodal age presentation, occurring in 3- to 4-month-old boys and in teenagers.[32,38] The embryonal type is the most common.

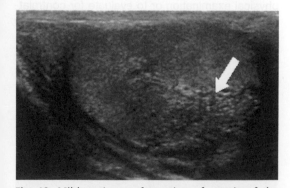

Fig. 19. Mild cystic transformation of ectasia of the rete testis in a 13-year-old boy found incidentally. Longitudinal scan of the right testis shows multiple circular structures in the posteromedial region extending to the mediastinum testis (*arrow*). There were also associated large spermatoceles (not shown).

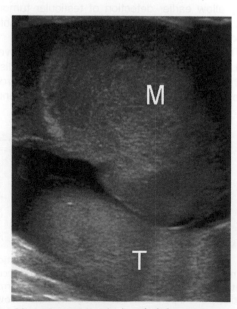

Fig. 20. Large paratesticular rhabdomyosarcoma in a 14-year-old boy. Longitudinal scan demonstrates the normal testis (T) and a large paratesticular mass (M).

These tumors can spread by hematogenous, lymphatic, and local routes. All patients should be evaluated for metastasis with liver function tests, bone scan, bone marrow aspirate, chest radiograph, and CT scan of the abdomen and pelvis. Radical inguinal orchiectomy is performed for all ages and stages. In boys younger than 10 years, retroperitoneal lymph node dissection is performed if there is imaging evidence of retroperitoneal lymphadenopathy. It is performed in all boys older than 10 years. The 3-year survival rate in all boys with paratesticular rhabdomyosarcoma is approximately 80%.[32]

There are benign extratesticular pathologies that can mimic tumors. These include hernia, hematoma, paratesticular fibrosis, and epididymitis (**Fig. 21**).[38]

CRYPTORCHYDISM

Cryptorchydism occurs in approximately 3% of term male infants with spontaneous descent in two-thirds of the cases. The incidence of cryptorchydism rises with prematurity because testicular descent usually occurs in the seventh month of gestation.[39,40]

Orchiopexy (surgery to place and fixate the gonad in the scrotum) prevents torsion of the cryptorchid testis and reduces the risk of trauma to the testis. The exact relationship of fertility to cryptorchydism and subsequent orchiopexy is controversial. Boys with cryptorchydism have increased risk of testicular cancer. Orchiopexy may allow earlier detection of testicular tumors, but it is controversial as to whether or not orchiopexy reduces the risk of testicular cancer.[41]

The role of US in guiding treatment is controversial. Some surgeons approach cryptorchydism without the guidance of US by performing laparoscopy and, if the laparoscopy is negative, continue

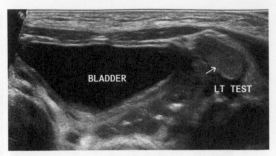

Fig. 22. Newborn with bilateral undescended testes. Transverse scan demonstrates a normal left testis (*arrow*) in the pelvis at the opening of the inguinal canal. The right testis was found in the same location.

with inguinal exploration.[39] Approximately 20% of undescended testes are nonpalpable and most of them are located in the inguinal canal (**Fig. 22**). US is highly sensitive for identifying the inguinal undescended testis. Using US to guide the surgical approach saves most boys from the need for laparoscopy.[40]

INGUINAL HERNIA AND HYDROCELE

Obliteration of the processus vaginalis occurs after the seventh month of gestation. Failure of the processus vaginalis to obliterate can result in passage of peritoneal fluid, leading to hydrocele or intestinal loops, or omentum, leading to inguinal hernia.[1–4,42]

The incidence of congenital inguinal hernia is between 0.8% and 4% of live births. The risk of incarceration is up to 60% in the first 6 months of life. Right inguinal hernias are more common as the right processus vaginalis closes later. In most cases, physical examination is sufficient for diagnosis. US can be helpful for inconclusive physical examination or to evaluate for contralateral involvement. US can show bowel loops in

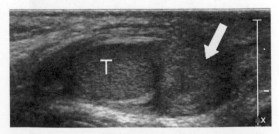

Fig. 21. Chronic epididymitis mimicking a paratesticular mass in a 2-year-old boy with epispadias and recurrent epididymitis. Longitudinal scan shows a normal testis (T) and a paratesticular echogenic mass (*arrow*). On exploration, a mass originated from the tail of the epididymis. Pathology demonstrated chronic inflammation.

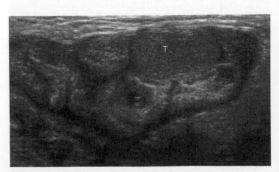

Fig. 23. Scrotal hernia in a 4-month-old boy. Longitudinal scan of the right scrotum demonstrates multiple bowel loops. Real-time scan demonstrated peristaltic activity. The testis (T) is normal.

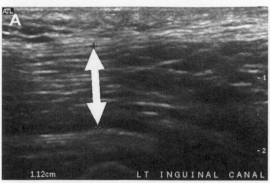
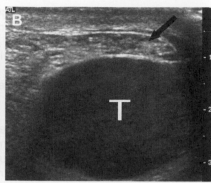

Fig. 24. Omental hernia in a 16-year-old boy. (*A*) Longitudinal scan of the left inguinal canal demonstrates marked widening (*double arrow*) of the inguinal canal with an echogenic material representing the omental hernia. (*B*) Longitudinal scan of the scrotum demonstrates the omentum extending to the scrotum (*arrow*). T, testis.

the inguinal canal or scrotum, and during real-time imaging it can demonstrate peristaltic activity or movement of fluid and air bubbles (**Fig. 23**). Omental hernia is seen as a continuous echogenic structure from the pelvis to the inguinal canal or scrotum (**Fig. 24**).

A clinically occult contralateral hernia can be found in 88% of cases. There is controversy about evaluation of occult contralateral inguinal hernia.[9,42] Some surgeons use visualization of the processus vaginalis with a laparoscope and others advocate evaluation by US. Demonstration of inguinal canal larger than 4 mm or containing fluid is an indication for prophylactic herniorrhaphy.[9]

Congenital hydrocele appears as fluid collection surrounding the anterolateral aspects of the testis, sometimes extending to the inguinal canal. When the processus vaginalis is completely patent, the hydrocele is communicating. This leads to elective repair. The processus vaginalis may obliterate at any point leading to various types of hydroceles. Closure of the processus vaginalis below the internal inguinal ring leads to noncommunicating

hydrocele, which usually resolves by the age of 1 year.[1–4,43]

Closure of the processus vaginalis below the internal inguinal ring and above the testis leads to spermatic cord hydrocele. A rare type of hydrocele is referred to as abdominoscrotal hydrocele. This is a large communicating hydrocele that protrudes through the internal inguinal ring into the abdominal cavity and appears as a pelvic cystic mass.

VARICOCELE

Dilatation of the pampiniform plexus in the scrotum is known as a varicocele. It results from incompetent gonadal veins. In the pediatric age group, varicocele most commonly presents in male adolescents and can cause pain and testicular hypoplasia. It is seen in approximately 15% of male adolescents and is 10 times more common in the left scrotum. Varicocele is usually diagnosed on physical examination of the warm, relaxed scrotum, with and without Valsalva maneuver, and with patients in the supine and upright position. Twenty-percent of male patients with

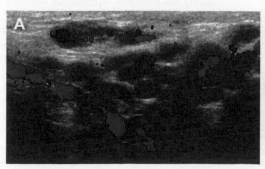
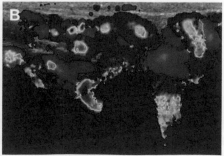

Fig. 25. Large left varicocele in a 13-year-old boy. (*A*) Color Doppler longitudinal scan demonstrates the plexus of distended veins in the left scrotum. (*B*) With Valsalva maneuver, the size of the varicocele increases maneuver.

varicocele have infertility, so the main challenge is to select patients who will benefit from treatment.[44,45]

US evidence of a varicocele is confirmed when serpentine vessels of the pampiniform plexus are greater than 2 mm in diameter and increase in size during Valsalva maneuver.[1–4] There are studies that show a potential role for duplex US in predicting the benefit of treatment in patients with veins having diameter of more than 3 mm,[46] higher retrograde flow,[47,48] and decreased volume of the testicle.[47] In addition, US can demonstrate varicoceles that are occult on physical examination of boys who may benefit from surgery.[49] US also serves to distinguish varicoceles from other causes of scrotal swelling, including hernias, hydroceles, and masses (**Fig. 25**).[1–4] Treatment options include varicocelectomy and percutaneous embolization of the gonadal veins.[44,45]

MICROLITHIASIS

Testicular microlithiases (TM) are calcifications surrounded by concentric layers of collagen fibers in the lumen of the seminiferous tubules. TM is uncommon and has been reported in 0.6% to 9% of adults. In US, TM is demonstrated as punctate echogenicities with a diameter of less than 3 mm and without shadowing.[50,51]

A study of 694 asymptomatic boys found a prevalence of classic microlithiasis (five or more echogenic foci) in 2.4% with increased prevalence with age.[52] It is most commonly idiopathic (**Fig. 26**). TM is described in association with various benign and malignant pathologies, including cryptorchydism, male pseudohermaphroditism, Klinefelter's syndrome, neurofibromatosis type 1, Down syndrome, varicocele, and germ cell tumors (see **Fig. 13**).[53–55]

There is no consensus on the risk of TM for development of testicular malignancy. Retro-

spective studies demonstrate the presence of microlithiasis in up to 40% of testicular malignancy. Prospective studies, however, do not show any increased risk in asymptomatic patients with testicular microlithiasis. It is, therefore, not clear if patients with idiopathic TM need to be followed by US.[50,51]

SUMMARY

Scrotal US is the preferred imaging for evaluation of scrotal pathologies. It is safe and readily available and provides high-resolution details. In addition, with the use of duplex US, perfusion can be assessed. Different pathologies of the scrotum may have the same clinical presentation and US is used to better define pathology and guide treatment. Routine scrotal US should include evaluation of the inguinal canals as it may improve detection of various scrotal pathologies, such as hernia, hydrocele, and testicular torsion.

REFERENCES

1. Dogra VS, Gottlieb RH, Oka M, et al. Sonography of the scrotum. Radiology 2003;227(1):18–36.
2. Aso C, Enríquez G, Fité M, et al. Gray-scale and color Doppler sonography of scrotal disorders in children: an update. Radiographics 2005;25(5):1197–214.
3. Munden MM, Trautwein LM. Scrotal pathology in pediatrics with sonographic imaging. Curr Probl Diagn Radiol 2000;29(6):185–205.
4. Hörmann M, Balassy C, Philipp MO, et al. Imaging of the scrotum in children. Eur Radiol 2004;14(6):974–83.
5. Kuijper EA, van Kooten J, Verbeke JI, et al. Ultrasonographically measured testicular volumes in 0- to 6-year-old boys. Humanit Rep 2008;23(4):792–6.
6. Hadziselimovic F, Zivkovic D, Bica DT, et al. The importance of mini-puberty for fertility in cryptorchidism. J Urol 2005;174:1536–9.
7. Raivio T, Toppari J, Keleva M, et al. Serum androgen bioactivity in cryptorchid and non-cryptorchid boys during the postnatal reproductive hormone surge. J Clin Endocrinol Metab 2003;88:2597–9.
8. Diamond DA, Paltiel HJ, DiCanzio J, et al. Comparative assessment of pediatric testicular volume: orchidometer versus ultrasound. J Urol 2000;164(3 Pt 2):1111–4.
9. Erez I, Rathause V, Vacian I, et al. Preoperative ultrasound and intraoperative findings of inguinal hernias in children: a prospective study of 642 children. J Pediatr Surg 2002;37(6):865–8.
10. McAndrew HF, Pemberton R, Kikiros CS, et al. The incidence and investigation of acute scrotal problems in children. Pediatr Surg Int 2002;18(5–6):435–7.

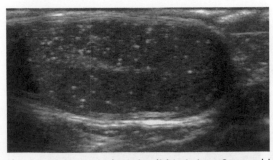

Fig. 26. Right testicular microlithiasis in a 6-year-old boy associated with left cryptorchydism. Longitudinal scan of the right testis demonstrates multiple diffuse non-shadowing echogenic foci in the testis.

11. Mäkelä E, Lahdes-Vasama T, Rajakorpi H, et al. A 19-year review of paediatric patients with acute scrotum. Scand J Surg 2007;96(1):62–6.

12. Kapoor S. Testicular torsion: a race against time. Int J Clin Pract 2008;62(5):821–7.

13. Karmazyn B, Steinberg R, Kornreich L, et al. Clinical and sonographic criteria of acute scrotum in children: a retrospective study of 172 boys. Pediatr Radiol 2005;35(3):302–10.

14. Kaye JD, Shapiro EY, Levitt SB, et al. Parenchymal echo texture predicts testicular salvage after torsion: potential impact on the need for emergent exploration. J Urol 2008;180(Suppl 4):1733–6.

15. Nussbaum Blask AR, Rushton HG. Sonographic appearance of the epididymis in pediatric testicular torsion. AJR 2006;187:1627–35.

16. Baud C, Veyrac C, Couture A, et al. Spiral twist of the spermatic cord: a reliable sign of testicular torsion. Pediatr Radiol 1998;28:950–3.

17. Arce JD, Cortes M, Vargas JC. Sonographic diagnosis of acute spermatic cord torsion. Rotation of the cord: a key to the diagnosis. Pediatr Radiol 2002;32:485–91.

18. Kalfa N, Veyrac C, Lopez M, et al. Multicenter assessment of ultrasound of the spermatic cord in children with acute scrotum. J Urol 2007;177(1):297–301.

19. Garel L, Dubois J, Azzie G, et al. Preoperative manual detorsion of the spermatic cord with Doppler ultrasound monitoring in patients with intravaginal acute testicular torsion. Pediatr Radiol 2000;30(1):41–4.

20. Sessions AE, Rabinowitz R, Hulbert WC, et al. Testicular torsion: direction, degree, duration and disinformation. J Urol 2003;169(2):663–5.

21. Traubici J, Daneman A, Navarro O. Original report. Testicular torsion in neonates and infants: sonographic features in 30 patients. AJR Am J Roentgenol 2003;180(4):1143–5.

22. Baldisserotto M, de Souza JC, Pertence AP, et al. Color Doppler sonography of normal and torsed testicular appendages in children. AJR Am J Roentgenol 2005;184(4):1287–92.

23. Karmazyn B, Steinberg R, Livne P, et al. Duplex sonographic findings in children with torsion of the testicular appendages: overlap with epididymitis and epididymoorchitis. J Pediatr Surg 2006;41(3):500–4.

24. Sakellaris GS, Charissis GC. Acute epididymitis in Greek children: a 3-year retrospective study. Eur J Pediatr 2008;167(7):765–9.

25. Merlini E, Rotundi F, Seymandi PL, et al. Acute epididymitis and urinary tract anomalies in children. Scand J Urol Nephrol 1998;32:273–5.

26. Siegel A, Snyder H, Duckett JW. Epididymitis in infants and boys: underlying urogenital anomalies and efficacy of imaging modalities. J Urol 1987;138:1100–3.

27. Cappèle O, Liard A, Barret E, et al. Epididymitis in children: is further investigation necessary after the first episode? Eur Urol 2000;38:627–30.

28. Karmazyn B, Kaefer M, Kauffman S, et al. Ultrasonography and clinical findings in children with epididymitis, with and without associated lower urinary tract abnormalities. Pediatr Radiol 2009;39:1054–8.

29. Lee A, Park SJ, Lee HK, et al. Acute idiopathic scrotal edema: ultrasonographic findings at an emergency unit. Eur Radiol 2009;19(8):2075–80.

30. Ross JH, Rybicki L, Kay R. Clinical behavior and a contemporary management algorithm for prepubertal testis tumors: a summary of the prepubertal testis tumor registry. J Urol 2002;168(4 Pt 2):1675–8 [discussion: 1678–9].

31. Aragona F, Pescatori E, Talenti E, et al. Painless scrotal masses in the pediatric population: prevalence and age distribution of different pathological conditions: a 10 year retrospective multicenter study. J Urol 1996;155(4):1424–6.

32. Agarwal PK, Palmer JS. Testicular and paratesticular neoplasms in prepubertal males. J Urol 2006;176(3):875–81.

33. Rubenstein RA, Dogra VS, Seftel AD, et al. Benign intrascrotal lesions. J Urol. 2004;171:1765–72.

34. Stikkelbroeck NM, Suliman HM, Otten BJ, et al. Testicular adrenal rest tumours in postpubertal males with congenital adrenal hyperplasia: sonographic and MR features. Eur Radiol 2003;13:1597–603.

35. Woodward PJ, Sohaey R, O'Donoghue MJ, et al. From the archives of the AFIP: tumors and tumorlike lesions of the testis: radiologic-pathologic correlation. Radiographics 2002;22(1):189–216.

36. Metcalfe PD, Farivar-Mohseni H, Farhat W, et al. Pediatric testicular tumors: contemporary incidence and efficacy of testicular preserving surgery. J Urol 2003;170(6 Pt 1):2412–5 [discussion: 2415–6].

37. Yossepowitch O, Karmazin B, Livne PM. Scrotal sonography for assisting in testis-sparing surgery in a prepubertal boy. AJR Am J Roentgenol 2001;176(6):1605–6.

38. Woodward PJ, Schwab CM, Sesterhenn IA. From the archives of the AFIP: extratesticular scrotal masses: radiologic-pathologic correlation. Radiographics 2003;23(1):215–40.

39. Elder JS. Ultrasonography is unnecessary in evaluating boys with a nonpalpable testis. Pediatrics 2002;110(4):748–51.

40. Nijs SM, Eijsbouts SW, Madern GC, et al. Nonpalpable testes: is there a relationship between ultrasonographic and operative findings? Pediatr Radiol 2007;37(4):374–9.

41. Wood HM, Elder JS. Cryptorchidism and testicular cancer: separating fact from fiction. J Urol 2009;181(2):452–61.

42. Rescorla FJ, West KW, Engum SA, et al. The "other side" of pediatric hernias: the role of laparoscopy. Am Surg 1997;63(8):690–3.

43. Wilson JM, Aaronson DS, Schrader R, et al. Hydrocele in the pediatric patient: inguinal or scrotal approach? J Urol 2008;180(Suppl 4):1724–7.

44. Kolon TF, Clement MR, Cartwright L, et al. Transient asynchronous testicular growth in adolescent males with a varicocele. J Urol 2008;180(3):1111–4.

45. Diamond DA, Zurakowski D, Bauer SB, et al. Relationship of varicocele grade and testicular hypotrophy to semen parameters in adolescents. J Urol 2007;178(4 Pt 2):1584–8.

46. Hussein AF. The role of color Doppler ultrasound in prediction of the outcome of microsurgical subinguinal varicocelectomy. J Urol 2006;176(5): 2141–5.

47. Kozakowski KA, Gjertson CK, Decastro GJ, et al. Peak retrograde flow: a novel predictor of persistent, progressive and new onset asymmetry in adolescent varicocele. J Urol 2009;181(6): 2717–22.

48. Schiff JD, Li PS, Goldstein M. Correlation of ultrasound- measured venous size and reversal of flow with Valsalva with improvement in semen-analysis parameters after varicocelectomy. Fertil Steril 2006; 86:250.

49. Jarow JP, Ogle SR, Eskew LA. Seminal improvement following repair of ultrasound detected subclinical varicoceles. J Urol 1996;155:1287.

50. Middleton WD, Teefey SA, Santillan CS. Testicular microlithiasis: prospective analysis of prevalence and associated tumor. Radiology 2002;224(2): 425–8.

51. Dagash H, Mackinnon EA. Testicular microlithiasis: what does it mean clinically? BJU Int 2007;99(1): 157–60.

52. Goede J, Hack WW, Voort-Doedens LM, et al. Prevalence of testicular microlithiasis in asymptomatic males 0 to 19 years old. J Urol 2009;182(4):1516–20.

53. Furness PD 3rd, Husmann DA, Brock JW 3rd, et al. Multi-institutional study of testicular microlithiasis in childhood: a benign or pre-malignant condition? J Urol 1998;160(3 Pt2):1151–4.

54. Kocaoğlu M, Bozlar U, Bulakbaşi N, et al. Testicular microlithiasis in pediatric age group: ultrasonography findings and literature review. Diagn Interv Radiol 2005;11(1):60–5.

55. Dell'Acqua A, Tomà P, Oddone M, et al. Testicular microlithiasis: US findings in six pediatric cases and literature review. Eur Radiol 1999;9(5):940–4.

Ultrasound of the Gastrointestinal Tract in the Neonate and Young Infant with Particular Attention to Problems in the Neonatal Intensive Care Unit

Kathleen M. McCarten, MD[a,b]

KEYWORDS

- Gastroesophageal reflux • Ultrasound bowel obstruction
- Ultrasound NEC • Prematures bowel perforation

OUTPATIENT UPPER GASTROINTESTINAL TRACT ULTRASOUND

Imaging of the gastrointestinal (GI) tract is usually considered within the realm of radiography and contrast fluoroscopy. The small size of newborns and small infants, however, allows evaluation by ultrasound. Usually the entire depth of the abdomen is within range of the transducer. Also, the types of abnormalities most commonly searched for are amenable to ultrasound evaluation and diagnosis. Bowel gas is a deterrent, but with graded compression, much of it may be displaced permitting deeper evaluation in the upper GI tract.

Pediatricians are commonly faced with the problem of a baby who is spitting up an excessive amount, which may be due to simple gastroesophageal reflux, but pyloric stenosis is often a concern. Similarly a baby who is colicky or constantly fussy may present a puzzle to a pediatrician especially in the situation of distraught and concerned young or first-time parents, and the pediatrician is hoping that the

solution may be as simple as reflux. The number of such patients can be large and overwhelm the limited resources of a small pediatric radiology department. At the author's institution, a screening abdominal ultrasound equivalent of an upper GI (UGI) is performed on all infants 4 months of age or younger who present with non-bilious vomiting, colic, fussiness, or question of pain and who are well appearing. If there are problems with feeding that suggest an esophageal or swallowing issue, such as gagging, coughing, or stridor, a traditional barium fluoroscopy examination is performed instead. In the circumstance of bilious vomiting or an infant who is ill, an abdominal ultrasound may be performed initially as part of the evaluation, but it is tailored to the particular clinical problem and combined with other imaging as needed, such as plain films to exclude bowel obstruction or contrast UGI if malrotation needs to be excluded (see the article by Cohen and colleagues elsewhere in this issue for further explanation of this topic). If an abnormality is discovered that

[a] Department of Radiology, The Warren Alpert Medical School of Brown University, 593 Eddy Street, Providence, RI 02903, USA
[b] Rhode Island Hospital, 593 Eddy Street, Providence, RI 02903, USA
E-mail address: KMcCarten@Lifespan.org

Ultrasound Clin 5 (2010) 75–95
doi:10.1016/j.cult.2009.11.010

cannot be completely delineated or answered by ultrasound, the baby is scheduled for a traditional barium study.

Infants are brought to the department after having fasted a normal feeding interval. The examination is performed using a high-frequency curved array transducer (range 6–8 MHz). A general evaluation of all of the major organs is performed to include liver, spleen, gallbladder, pancreas, adrenals, kidneys, and large vascular structures to assure normalcy. The normal relationship of the mesenteric vessels is documented. The normal relationship is that the superior mesenteric vein (SMV) is anterior and to the right of the superior mesenteric artery (SMA). This normal relationship, however, does not totally exclude malrotation (discussed later).

Hypertrophic Pyloric Stenosis and Gastric Outlet Obstruction

In performing an examination for pyloric stenosis, the author uses the method described by Teele and Share[1] in placing an infant supine on an examining table with a towel rolled under the left side such that the infant is lying in a right posterior oblique position. Although pyloric stenosis may not be present, in its absence the examination is carried further to evaluate the entire duodenum. A high-frequency linear array transducer (range 9–12 MHz) is used to locate the antrum and pylorus by identifying the gallbladder and moving slightly medially. The infant is then offered a bottle to drink in this position.

A 5% dextrose and water solution is the ideal choice; 30 to 60 mL is usually sufficient (**Fig. 1**). Administering too much fluid overdistends the stomach, and the antrum and pylorus may rotate posteriorly and become more difficult to visualize. If the referring clinician has prescribed Pedialyte (Abbott Nutrition, Columbus, OH, USA) or another electrolyte solution due to excessive vomiting, this can be used as an alternative. By ultrasound, Pedialyte sometimes appears clear like sugar water or can have a more echogenic appearance, because, with turbulence, it may acquire an effervescent character (personal observation) (**Fig. 2**).

At times some infants are reluctant to drink from a type of bottle provided by the hospital that is dissimilar to what is usually used; in this circumstance, the fluid can be placed into the infant's own bottle for more comfort. Breastfed babies who have never been fed by bottle may be reluctant to feed from a bottle and in these circumstances the infant can be breastfed and then placed on the examining table for evaluation. Although not as echolucent as sugar water, breast milk is usually uniform enough that the examination is satisfactory. If an infant has been fasting, even formula can function as an appropriate agent. When imaging is performed immediately after the fluid is given, it is still uniform and not curdled, and may sometimes outline the duodenal sweep better than other materials.

By placing a baby in the steep right posterior oblique position, the ingested fluid preferentially flows to the antrum, which becomes better identified when distended by fluid. Normal antral and

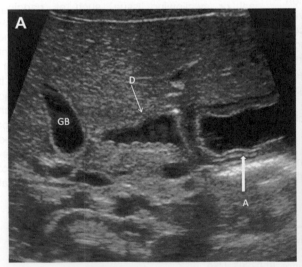
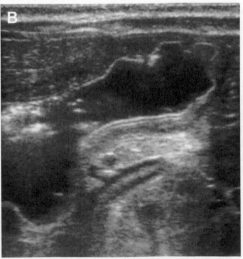

Fig. 1. Normal duodenum and stomach. (*A*) The duodenum (D) and antrum of the stomach (A) are normally distended with fluid. The gall bladder (GB) is seen adjacent to the duodenum. (*B*) Normally distended body and fundus of stomach.

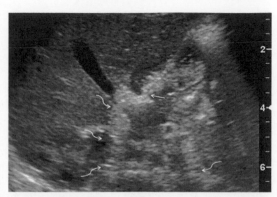

Fig. 2. Normal pylorus. Effervescent Pedialyte is seen passing through the pylorus (*straight arrow*) and extending around the entire C-loop of the duodenum (*curved arrows*).

pyloric wall thickness measures approximately 2 to 3 mm.[2,3] If pyloric stenosis is present, it is easily seen. If pyloric stenosis is present, the stomach is frequently seen to be fluid filled despite a normal fasting period and no further fluid need be given. Care must be taken to observe for a sufficient amount of time to differentiate severe pyloro-spasm from true pyloric stenosis.

Other gastric abnormalities may be encountered, such as gastric duplication, antral webs, or focal alveolar hyperplasia (seen in babies on prostaglandin therapy to maintain patency of the ductus arteriosus in duct dependent congenital heart disease) (**Fig. 3**).[4,5]

Once a normal antrum has been outlined, the fluid is then observed passing through the pylorus into the duodenum, filling a normal-shaped

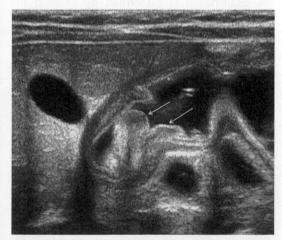

Fig. 3. Foveolar hyperplasia. Longitudinal sonogram of the gastric antrum and pylorus shows two protuberant mounds of mucosal tissue in the gastric antrum (*arrows*), which proved to be foveolar hyperplasia at biopsy.

duodenal bulb and descending duodenum. The presence of pylorospasm may require patience to allow for the pylorus to relax and allow fluid to pass. Abnormalities, such as duodenal webs, duodenal stenosis, duodenal duplication (**Fig. 4**), or annular pancreas, can be identified. To and fro peristalsis is an ancillary finding of proximal bowel obstruction. This can be visualized by ultrasound in the same fashion in which it is seen fluoroscopically.

Malrotation

As with a barium study, the endpoint of any UGI should be documenting a normal ligament of Treitz in an attempt to exclude malrotation. To better visualize the transverse duodenum, the baby is changed to a flat supine position and the pancreas visualized transversely. The fluid in the stomach may actually aid in visualizing the entire pancreas. If there is a large amount of gastric air present from feeding, the baby can be burped and the examination continued. Slow compression can be used to displace gas in the obscuring bowel loops. The mesenteric vessels are again observed to document the normal relationship of the SMV slightly anterior and to the right of the SMA. Although a normal relationship does not exclude malrotation, it suggests that this abnormality is unlikely. If the relationship is abnormal, further evaluation of the transverse duodenum is performed, but depending on whether or not an unequivocal identification is made, a radiographic UGI may then be scheduled to confirm without question, the presence or absence of malrotation. One series found that UGI and ultrasound were both normal in 62% of their cases, both abnormal in 15%, false positive in 21% where the ultrasound was abnormal but the UGI was normal, and 2% false where the ultrasound was interpreted as normal but the UGI was abnormal.[6]

After the mesenteric vessels are identified, the transducer is moved a small amount caudally to visualize the fluid traveling through the transverse duodenum as it passes under the SMA and crosses the midline to the left. This is the most difficult and challenging portion of the examination, requires patience and practice for proficiency, and can become time intensive. It is an observation more easily made in real time than on static images (**Fig. 5**).

At times, if the baby is relaxed and there is little bowel gas present, compression may used to identify the transverse duodenum even without the presence of fluid (**Fig. 5B**). Large amounts of air in colon are the most common reason for this portion of the examination to be

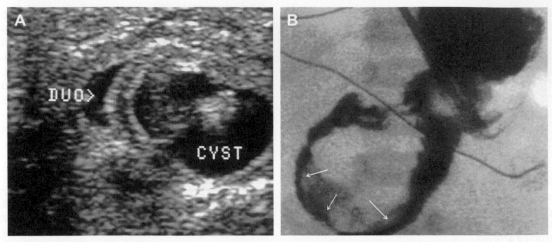

Fig. 4. Duplication cyst. (A) Transverse sonogram shows fluid in the duodenal lumen (DUO) compressed by a duplication cyst (CYST) that contains some debris. (B) The corresponding fluoroscopic UGI image demonstrates extrinsic compression and narrowing of the lumen of the entire duodenal C-loop (*arrows*).

unsuccessful. Consequently, if there is any continued concern for malrotation or other distal duodenal abnormality, a formal barium examination is indicated.

Recently it has been suggested that not only is the relationship between the SMA and the SMV not reliable but that a UGI may demonstrate false-positive and false-negative appearances if only the position of the duodenojejunal junction is considered; in other words, a ligament of Treitz that is considered too low radiographically may be normal and one that is in the expected position may be abnormal. This presentation states that the only essential finding needed to exclude malrotation is that the third portion of the duodenum be retromesenteric.[7] This is the relationship that the

author's institution strives to identify in all of examinations. A more thorough discussed of malrotation is included in the article by Cohen and colleagues elsewhere in this issue.

Gastroesophageal Reflux

Gastroesophageal reflux is a common occurrence in young infants. Under most circumstances it resolves spontaneously with time and can be treated symptomatically if there are not superimposed problems, such as failure to thrive, significant esophagitis, or aspiration. The extent of evaluation of reflux by ultrasound varies with the complexity of the clinical problem. This portion of the examination is performed by keeping the

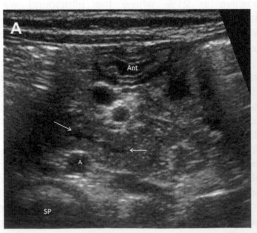
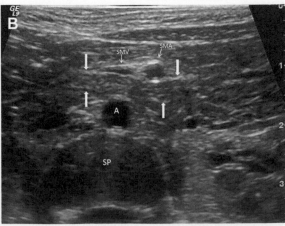

Fig. 5. Normal duodenal rotation (A) Transverse sonogram shows fluid passing through the lumen of the transverse duodenum (*arrows*) anterior to the spine (SP) and aorta (A) and posterior to the normally positioned mesenteric vessels and antrum (Ant) of the stomach. (B) The duodenum (*outlined by arrows*) is compressed without fluid in its lumen, but the redundancy of the duodenal folds can be seen passing behind the SMV and SMA.

baby supine in a flat position and placing the linear array transducer in a craniocaudad plane over the left lobe of the liver just to the left of midline. The air or fluid in the fundus of the stomach can be localized and the transducer can then be moved slowly medially in a slight oblique orientation with the craniad end of the transducer angled slightly toward the right until the lower esophagus and gastroesophageal junction are located. The appearance of the normal lower esophagus is that of parallel hypoechoic walls and more echogenic mucosa. A stripe of intraluminal air can help to identify it (**Fig. 6**).

Having a baby swallow a small amount of fluid under observation can help localize the esophagus if there is difficulty otherwise. In order to visualize reflux, observation can be performed for a selected period of time with the transducer positioned over the gastroesophageal junction. If more accurate evaluation for an individual patient is desired, an infant can at this point in the examination be given as much fluid as is normally given in a feeding and then further observation performed. Under real-time observation the gastroesophageal junction is seen to open and gastric fluid reflux into the esophagus (**Fig. 7**). Although hiatal hernias are rare in small infants, their presence can be detected (**Fig. 8**).

Rather than a linear column of fluid or air refluxing through the gastroesophageal junction, dilatation of the distal esophagus is visualized using the

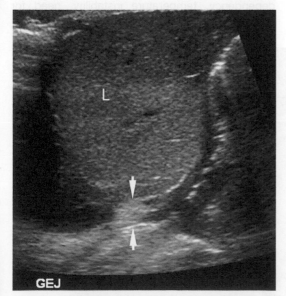

Fig. 6. Gastroesophageal junction. Longitudinal sonogram shows the closed gastroesophageal junction (*arrows*) seen through the liver (L) with a minimal amount of air outlining its margin.

liver as an acoustic window. Confirmation and better definition can then be performed using a traditional barium study (**Fig. 8**B).

Using ultrasound to identify reflux is well described in the literature but there are also objections, indicating that the height of the reflux cannot be determined and that should aspiration occur, this would not be detected. Similarly, ultrasound would not detect reflux that occurs in the interval between feedings. It does, however, detect reflux that is sustained with dilatation. If multiple episodes of reflux are seen in a short period of time without frank vomiting, this may allow an explanation for irritability or esophagitis. As discussed previously, the author's institution uses this study as a screening examination that may then lead to tailored follow-up studies. A more invasive modality is 24-hour pH probe placement to more accurately identify numbers of episodes of reflux.[8] More detail than just the presence or absence of reflux may be desired. Some investigators have described specific angles measured between the esophagus and stomach, a beak configuration to the gastroesophageal junction, or a shorter than normal intra-abdominal segment of stomach.[9,10]

GASTROINTESTINAL ULTRASOUND IN THE NEONATAL ICU

Advances in management have allowed the survival of premature infants born at progressively earlier gestational ages. In recent years there has been an increase in the number of premature births, much of which is related to multiple gestation pregnancies, particularly from in vitro fertilization. This has resulted in many neonatal ICUs (NICUs) having an increased number of very low-birth-weight (VLBW) infants less than 1500 g and extremely low-birth-weight (ELBW) infants of less than 1000 g. Advances in monitoring and support equipment have increased the survival of more of these fragile babies. In the author's NICU, the survival rate of babies 750 g or less was 45% in 1995; in 2009 the survival for the same-sized baby at 750 g or less is greater than 90% (James Padbury, MD, personal communication).

GI disorders seen in NICUs are congenital or acquired. The congenital abnormalities are usually obstructive in nature and often have been recognized by prenatal ultrasound or MRI. In the absence of any prenatal imaging, obstructive lesions are suspected by clinical presentation and radiographic imaging. Acquired disorders usually relate to prematurity and its complications. Each of these two types of processes has a different set of issues, but the imaging approach is similar. Birth weight and gestational age dictate

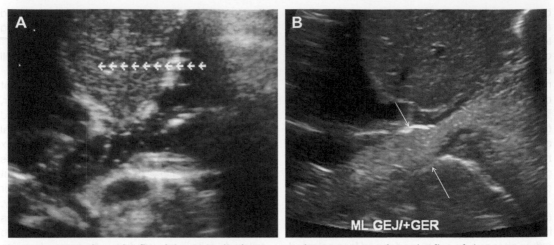

Fig. 7. Gastroesophageal reflux. (*A*) Longitudinal sonogram shows gastroesophageal reflux of clear sugar water with the direction confirmed by arrows. (*B*) This baby had been given formula, which is more echogenic but nonetheless demonstrates the reflux well (*arrows*).

management and tailor, which imaging examinations are feasible. These are discussed in detail.

Plain film radiography is the principle modality for abdominal imaging in NICUs. The evaluation of intestinal gas patterns and distinction of normal from pathologic can be crucial. The normal radiographic appearance of the abdomen is of diffuse, even distribution of bowel gas throughout the abdomen. Normal bowel presents a polyhedral configuration with only the thickness of normal bowel wall separating the gas of two adjacent loops. The only loop that should have any appearance of being at all elongated is colon. Colon

cannot always be differentiated from small bowel but if necessary a prone view may demonstrate gas in the rectum if it is not apparent on the supine examination to document the contiguity of the GI tract.

Bowel distension in particular may have myriad causes, some of which may be treated by conservative measures whereas others may require more drastic measures, including surgery. Multiple factors prevent tiny premature infants from being moved out of a neonatal unit for fluoroscopic investigation of GI problems, including ventilator dependency, temperature instability, need for

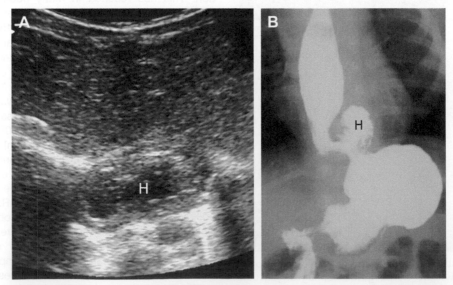

Fig. 8. Hiatal hernia. (*A*) Transverse image of the upper abdomen shows a distended fluid-filled hiatal hernia (H) in the midline posterior to the liver. (*B*) This finding was confirmed on a subsequent barium UGI.

careful body temperature monitoring, vulnerability to excessive handling, insensible fluid loss, hypotension, and electrolyte imbalance secondary to contrast administration. Because of these considerations, it is impractical to transport ill premature newborns, especially ELBW infants, out of the more stable confines of a well-managed NICU. Thus, it is vital that all diagnostic studies be performed within NICUs, and beyond the information obtained from radiography, the major viable alternative is ultrasound.

General Approach to the Neonatal ICU Patient

Most examinations are performed using a high-frequency linear array transducer with a range of 4 to 9 MHz with additional functions of pulse subtraction harmonics and differential tissue harmonics, which aid in achieving superb detail. In addition, a smaller "hockey stick" transducer may be used, with a range of 7 to 14 MHz. This probe, which is normally indicated for small parts and superficial structures, functions well even for the entire abdominal examination in VLBW or ELBW infants (**Fig. 9**). It serves also as an ancillary tool in circumstances in which there are multiple catheters, tubes, or monitoring devices covering a large amount of the surface of a small abdomen, allowing a sonographer the ability to circumvent these devices to complete a thorough examination. The smaller transducer also allows evaluation of small vascular structures when there is concern for thrombosis.

As with any complete abdominal examination, the solid organs are inspected first, including the liver, spleen, gallbladder and biliary tract, pancreas, adrenal glands, kidneys, and urinary bladder. Major vascular structures are identified: aorta and its larger branches, such as the celiac axis, SMA, and renal arteries; inferior vena cava; hepatic veins, and the portal venous system. The presence or absence of free fluid is confirmed and, if present, its character is noted.

Nasogastric suction is used frequently to put the GI tract at rest and to decompress the air that may be introduced with ventilation for concomitant lung disease. A stomach and intestinal tract void of gas allows easier ultrasound visualization. The small size of the neonate and the closeness of all of the intra-abdominal structures to the skin surface permits exquisite imaging detail of mural and mucosal components of stomach or bowel. A transverse ultrasonographic image of the upper abdomen often resembles an axial CT image of the upper abdomen in an older child or adult (**Fig. 10**). The presence of gastric and bowel gas produces more of a challenge, but graded compression or evaluation from flank or through a fluid filled urinary bladder many times allows more optimal visualization and alleviates the problem.

Congenital Abnormalities

Congenital abnormalities are comprised primarily of obstructive lesions, structural or functional. Plain film radiography and contrast fluoroscopy are the workhorse studies in evaluation of these entities. The radiography of congenital GI abnormalities are well described in several pediatric

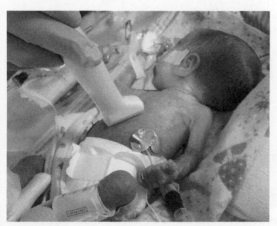

Fig. 9. Examination technique. Photo of a 710-g premature infant illustrating the relative size of the 14-MHz probe normally used for small part examinations.

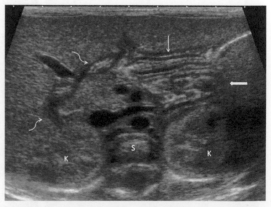

Fig. 10. Normal anatomy. Transverse image of the upper abdomen in a 350-g infant with an appearance similar to an axial CT image (K, kidney; S, spine). Gastric antral wall (*straight narrow arrow*) duodenal sweep (*curved arrows*), and proximal jejunal loops (*broad arrow*).

radiology texts and well summarized in an article by Hernanz-Schulman.[11] For pediatric surgeons, the maximum amount of information available before surgery may alter the approach and prevent surprises of discovery of unexpected abnormalities once the surgical procedure is underway. Because of the fragile nature of small premature infants, the shortest surgical procedure time feasible is mandatory. Plain radiographs are the usual initial imaging examination performed. The information gained from these and that obtained from prenatal studies often indicates a specific abnormality. Significant prematurity or endotracheal intubation may preclude immediate postnatal evaluation by fluoroscopic studies. In these circumstances an abdominal ultrasound substantiates the features diagnosed prenatally and may add considerably more information. If no prenatal studies were performed and the cause of the problem is unknown, a full evaluation is indicated. The diagnostic ability and experience of the physician performing the examination and the confidence of the surgeon in the findings obtained may preclude the need for further radiographic studies preoperatively. Efficiency in performing the examination is also essential if an infant's clinical status is unstable; assistance by a nurse or neonatologist may be required.

Duodenal obstruction

Duodenal atresia has the classic plain film radiographic appearance of a double bubble due to a dilated stomach and proximal duodenum. Of all patients with duodenal atresia, 30% to 40% have trisomy 21 and, in infants with trisomy 21, 15% have duodenal atresia.[11–13] It is the most common location for atresia. In the usual situation, no further imaging is needed and an infant is brought to the operating room for definitive repair. If, however, surgery needs to be delayed secondary to other medical problems, such as coexistent lung or cardiac disease, abdominal ultrasound should be performed to exclude malrotation. Malrotation has been reported to occur in 28% of neonates with duodenal atresia.[14] Several sources suggest that the only indication for ultrasound evaluation in duodenal atresia is the coexistence of esophageal atresia without a distal fistula,[15] in which case there is no gas in the stomach and all evaluation needs to be performed by ultrasound. If, however, malrotation needs to be excluded, ultrasound is the only easily accessible alternative. As with the normal UGI, the mesenteric vessels are identified. The proximal duodenum is dilated and frequently fluid filled, allowing easy visualization. It then can be followed to its termination at the atretic level or narrowing, in the case of duodenal stenosis. Moving progressively medially with the transducer, a collapsed distal duodenum passing posterior to the mesenteric vessels and extending toward the duodenojejunal junction can be identified (**Fig. 11**).

Other entities can cause duodenal obstruction. Annular pancreas can occur alone or can be

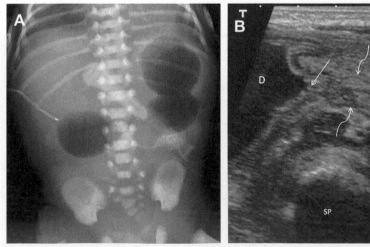

Fig. 11. Duodenal atresia. (A) Supine radiograph of the abdomen shows the classic double bubble appearance. (B) Transverse sonogram demonstrates some fluid in the dilated duodenum (D) with the point of narrowing shown with a straight arrow. Distal to the atresia a collapsed duodenum is seen (*curved arrows*) passing between the mesenteric vessels (smv and sma) and the aorta (A), which is anterior to the spine (SP). This confirms the absence of associated malrotation.

associated with duodenal atresia[12] and also can be diagnosed with preoperative ultrasound examination. Duodenal webs can be identified, particularly by giving clear fluid to the infant to outline the dilated proximal duodenum. Depending on the degree of obstruction, the fluid may be seen passing into smaller caliber distal duodenum or may demonstrate to and fro peristalsis.

Duplication cysts of the GI tract can occur anywhere along the GI tract but most often in the ileum.[15] These often present later in infancy or childhood. Duodenal duplication cysts occur less frequently, representing approximately 2% to 12% of duplications, but these present earlier and have even been reported prenatally.[14] They form along the mesenteric border of the first or second portion of the duodenum and thus are accessible to identification (see **Fig. 4**). Characteristics include a typical muscular appearance to the wall; the cyst is often filled with debris.[16]

Small bowel obstruction

Bowel atresias beyond the duodenum are due to vascular insults causing previously intact bowel to necrose and subsequently compromise the bowel lumen. Jejunal or ileal atresias occur in 1 per 3000 live births. Jejunal atresias tend to be multiple and the jejunum has greater capacity to dilate before a perforation occurs. Ileal atresias tend to be solitary and perforation occurs more readily with little dilatation.[12] Some investigators believe that ultrasound is not helpful preoperatively[15] but at the author's institution the approach is different. Plain radiographs document that an obstruction exists requiring surgery. If only a proximal small bowel atresia is present, the caliber of the colon may still be normal due to the fluid and succus entericus produced by small bowel. A more distal small bowel atresia is associated with a microcolon because the colon has never been stimulated to develop because of the lack of passage of bowel contents. The diagnosis of microcolon is usually made by contrast enema but can be made by ultrasound evaluation. Similarly, an overall approximation of total bowel caliber can be made as can the relative number of dilated loops versus decompressed postobstructive segments. Although a surgeon may want to confirm findings by contrast enema before surgical intervention, if the neonate is unstable, preliminary evaluation by ultrasound may allow sufficient baseline information to more comfortably delay surgery until the clinical situation stabilizes.

The approach to a patient with a high-grade obstruction is to systematically evaluate the bowel segments. Malrotation with volvulus can be associated with atresia and can first be excluded by evaluation of the mesenteric vessels to be certain that there is no volvulus or "swirl" sign (see the article by Cohen and colleagues elsewhere in this issue for further explanation of this topic). The extent of dilated bowel loops is then determined. At times, the focus of obstruction can be identified (**Fig. 12**), particularly if the number of dilated fluid filled loops is not too numerous. An estimation of the extent of decompressed loops distal to an obstruction can be made. Decompressed small bowel loops distal to atretic bowel loops are easily identifiable (**Fig. 13**). Because of the fixed location of segments of colon, they are usually easy to follow. The retroperitoneal location of ascending and descending colon allows visualization by scanning with a linear array transducer along each flank in a craniocaudad direction. Even in the presence of dilated small bowel, an almost lateral approach virtually always allows visualization of ascending and descending colon. The transverse colon is less easily followed along its course as dilated small bowel may obscure it. The rectum in a neonate is easily identifiable transabdominally. The small anterior posterior diameter of a newborn pelvis permits adequate penetration of the pelvic structures by the transducer such that the sacrum can be easily identified with the rectum anterior to it. A fluid-filled urinary bladder or the relatively large neonatal uterus may provide an acoustic window and may help to demonstrate it more clearly. The caliber of colon can be compared with small bowel to make a determination of microcolon in a similar fashion to the way in which it is evaluated by contrast enema. When there is decompressed colon or microcolon, the rectum can be followed retrograde with the transducer to its junction with the descending colon.

Meconium ileus versus atresia

Fluid in bowel proximal to a simple atresia has the characteristic appearance of particles freely mobile within the fluid filled dilated loops. With real-time observation, the movement of the intraluminal fluid is easily identifiable. This is in contradistinction to meconium ileus where the bowel contents are thick and change little with observation, pressure, or movement.[17] Meconium ileus may be associated with atresia, which causes bowel distension proximally[13] or may produce bowel dilatation by developing inspissated meconium primarily in distal small bowel. Distinguishing simple bowel atresia from meconium ileus with atresia or meconium ileus without atresia alters subsequent management. If there is meconium ileus without atresia and inspissated material is

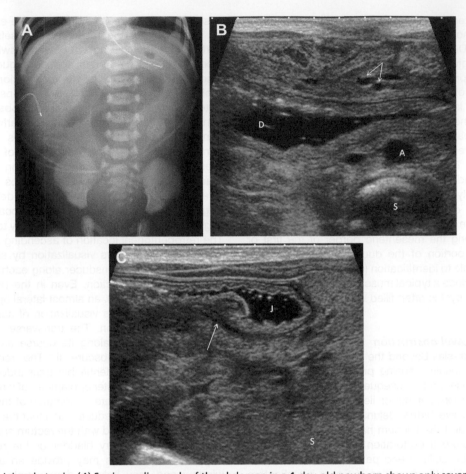

Fig. 12. Jejunal atresia. (*A*) Supine radiograph of the abdomen in a 1-day-old newborn shows only several dilated loops of proximal bowel. (*B*) Transverse sonogram shows a distended duodenum (D) passing between the mesenteric vessels (*arrows*) and the aorta (A) in front of the spine (S). (*C*) The duodenum could then be followed to the proximal jejunum (J) to the point of atresia (*arrow*).

seen to extend into distal small bowel, attempts may be made to evacuate the bowel contents by performing contrast enemas rather than subjecting an infant to immediate surgery. Because 15% of newborns with cystic fibrosis have meconium ileus as their presenting symptom,[12] any finding to aid in early definitive diagnosis may be helpful to clinicians and families.

Meconium peritonitis
Prenatal bowel perforation causes meconium to come in contact with peritoneum producing a chemical peritonitis. This results in calcification, which has been shown by prenatal ultrasound to occur rapidly. A prenatal diagnosis warrants postnatal evaluation. The clinical situation postnatally can vary considerably. The neonate may be completely asymptomatic if there was a single localized perforation that sealed off or could present with bowel

obstruction due to the underlying cause of the perforation (ie, malrotation, atresia, meconium ileus, and so forth).

Initial evaluation is by plain radiograph. In the situation of localized sealed off perforation, the bowel gas pattern may be normal with the only positive finding being peritoneal calcifications. In more extensive perforation, there may be diffuse calcification, clustered calcification in a localized meconium "cyst," or even calcifications in the scrotum by extension through the processus vaginalis. Diffuse shadowing calcific densities may be seen studding the peritoneal surface, an appearance sometimes referred to as a "snowstorm." It is not only the presence of meconium peritonitis that is of interest to surgeons but also information that can be obtained as to the cause. The goal of ultrasound is to evaluate for cause and complications of perforation. A calcified wall of a mass may be identified, and bowel may be incorporated

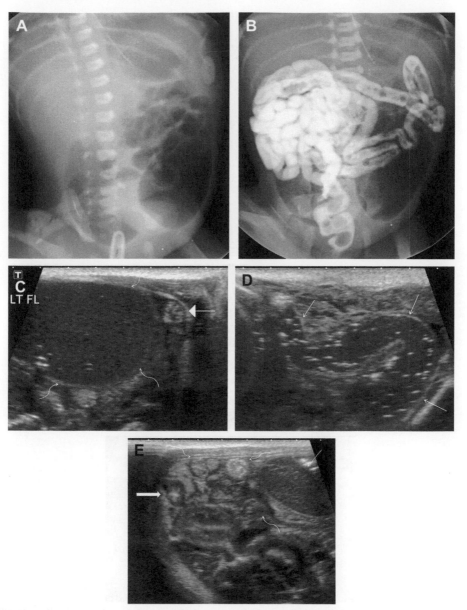

Fig. 13. Ileal atresia. (*A*) Supine radiograph shows more loops of bowel are visualized than in jejunal atresia, with varying degrees of distension. (*B*) Contrast enema shows the small-sized colon and nondilated distal small bowel loops. (*C*) Ultrasound image along the left flank include the very dilated bowel loop (*curved arrows*) and adjacent to it the small caliber descending colon (*broad arrow*). (*D*) A less dilated fluid filled loop is outlined by straight arrows. (*E*) Small bowel loops of normal to small caliber (*curved arrows*) are seen distal to the level of obstruction and adjacent to a small ascending colon (*broad arrow*).

into the mass. At times the density of the intraperitoneal meconium at sonography may not appear as dense as expected from radiographs (see **Fig. 14**).[18,19,20]

Hirschsprung's disease

The hallmark of diagnosing Hirschsprung's disease is documenting a transition zone between dilated proximal colon and more narrow distal colon or rectum. A transition zone in the rectosigmoid region accounts for 90% of cases.[11] Failure to pass stool normally and radiographs demonstrating diffuse distension, including colon, lead to evaluation. Often the diagnosis can be suspected on plain radiograph but contrast enema is the usual next study. As with plain films or contrast enemas, the transition zone can be identified by ultrasound. In the same manner as described previously in evaluating for microcolon, the

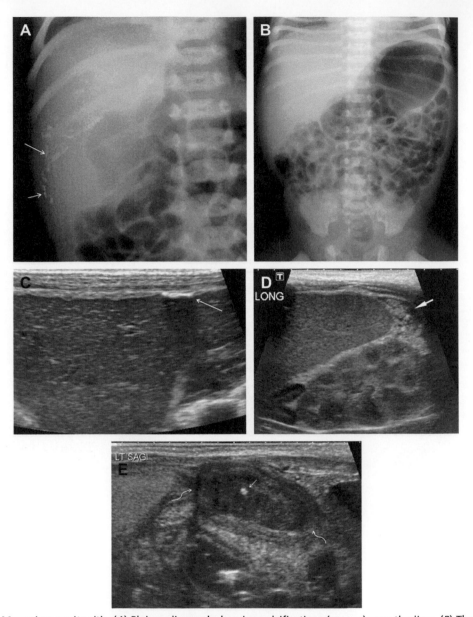

Fig. 14. Meconium peritonitis. (*A*) Plain radiograph showing calcifications (*arrows*) over the liver. (*B*) The normal bowel gas pattern indicates an intrauterine perforation that sealed off resulting in no long-term sequelae. (*C*) Sonogram along the liver margin shows shadowing calcifications (*arrow*). (*D*) Ill-defined but not yet calcified debris (*arrow*) can be seen surrounding the tip of the liver. (*E*) In another patient, a small meconium cyst is seen (*curved arrows*) with a small internal calcification (*straight arrow*).

ascending colon is outlined by following its course along the right flank. Whether or not filled with air or fecal material, its diameter can be measured. Similarly, the descending colon can be followed along its course and its diameter measured in transverse diameter. The rectum is then identified and its transverse diameter measured and then compared with ascending and descending colon to evaluate for change in caliber (**Fig. 15**). As with contrast enemas, equal

calibers throughout suggest absence of Hirschsprung's; in this situation, a decision can be made not to perform a rectal biopsy to evaluate for ganglion cells immediately but to follow clinically. A definite transition zone, or even an equivocal one, warrants biopsy for confirmation.

Meconium plug and small left colon
Meconium plug and small left colon are two entities that may be variations of the same process.

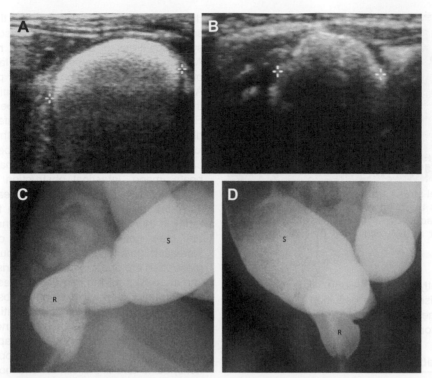

Fig. 15. Hirschsprung's disease. (*A*) Transverse sonogram shows a dilated sigmoid colon (calipers) compared with (*B*), a much smaller rectum (calipers) in an image done at the same degree of magnification. (*C*) Lateral and (*D*) anteroposterior fluoroscopic views of the distal colon confirms the ultrasound findings, showing the transition form a dilated sigmoid (S) to a small rectum (R). Hirschsprung's disease was confirmed by rectal biopsy.

Normal meconium may get "stuck" along its course through the colon frequently at the level of the splenic flexure. Small left colon is an entity seen frequently in infants of diabetic mothers that may represent immature function of colon preventing normal passage of meconium immediately after birth. The clinical presentation of a full term neonate with bowel distension that extends distally into colon and with little or no passage of meconium suggests the diagnosis. There is, however, considerable overlap in the appearance of obstructive or functional disorders, and a specific diagnosis cannot be made on plain radiograph. Because contrast enema may be therapeutic and diagnostic, it is often the next indicated procedure. Some investigators feel that ultrasound may be helpful. Couture[13] has shown that in the small left colon syndrome, ultrasound demonstrates that the descending colon has a small caliber relative to the transverse or ascending colon but, unlike in Hirschsprung's disease, the caliber of the rectum is normal.

Anal atresia
Diagnosis of anal atresia is clinically obvious at birth but the entity requires further investigation from several different aspects. Because anal atresia may be part of the vertebral, anal atresia, tracheoesophageal atresia, renal, cardiac, limb complex of abnormalities, surveillance for associated abnormalities includes renal and spine ultrasound. Although bony abnormalities of the spine may be evident by ultrasound, radiographic evaluation is indicated for complete evaluation.

Of more importance is the establishment of the level of atresia, whether or not low below the rectal muscular sling or high terminating above the sling. The level has totally different surgical implications with high atresias requiring more extensive surgical procedures. Plain radiographs are imprecise in establishing the level. Ultrasound from the perineal approach can identify the distance between the skin surface and the distal tip of the rectal pouch. Most sources report that a distance of less than 1 to 1.5 cm indicates a low lesion and a distance of greater than 1.5 cm indicates a high lesion.[15,21] Some investigators use ultrasound to distinguish the individual muscles in the puborectal sling allowing more definitive diagnosis of high versus low atresia.[22] In all male infants with high atresia, there is an obligatory rectovesical fistula present, which may be identifiable by ultrasound confirming a high atresia (**Fig. 16**). This can be evaluated

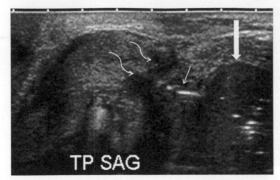

Fig. 16. Anal atresia. Longitudinal transperineal sonogram shows the blind ending rectum of a high anal atresia (*broad arrow*) with a small fistula containing air (*straight arrow*) leading to the urethra (*curved arrows*).

subsequently by fluoroscopy with contrast for more precise anatomic definition preoperatively. MRI has the ability to define the muscle groups of the levator sling for more accurate evaluation.[23]

Acquired abnormalities

Structural abnormalities of the GI tract (described previously) most often lead to a surgical procedure with ultrasound providing optimal anatomic detail and thus a more precise road map for surgeons. Medical problems that develop, particularly in the small premature infant, often create a more difficult clinical situation for neonatologists. Any substantive addition to the clinical picture that can be added by imaging can alter management.

Most admissions to NICUs are for prematurity and its related respiratory problems, which often require long-term endotracheal intubation. This in itself interferes with normal feeding and nutrition but when the GI tract is also immature, feeding, nutrition, and growth are problematic. Vascular access catheters, endotracheal tubes, enteric tubes, and simple handling all add potential sources of infection and complications that affect multiple organ systems, including the GI tract.

Some of the common clinical problems that arise in NICUs include abdominal distension, increased gastric residuals, or bilious aspirates. Any of these symptoms may be benign and transient but vigilance is indicated to exclude the development of a more ominous condition, such as obstruction or necrotizing enterocolitis (NEC). Imaging is vital in this differentiation. Abdominal distension can be a result of factors as simple as gas introduced with continuous positive airway pressure, producing diffuse gaseous bowel

distension from stomach to rectum that is easily seen on plain radiographs. Ileus associated with systemic stress or sepsis may be responsible. Ascites, hepatosplenomegaly, and a large amount of free air from perforation are other possibilities. Ascites can be suspected from plain films but the character of the fluid cannot be discerned. Hepatosplenomegaly can be inferred from displacement of the bowel gas in the expected location of the organs. Free intraperitoneal air can be diagnosed with an additional horizontal beam image. Intestinal obstruction can cause bowel distension or can result in increased gastric aspirates or bilious aspirates. Plain film radiography in this situation may support the possibility but may not indicate a cause or location. Increased gastric aspirates or bilious aspirates most often are due to diminished peristalsis of an immature GI tract but can be the presenting sign of malrotation and volvulus, other obstruction, or NEC. Plain film diagnosis of malrotation alone or malrotation with volvulus usually is not possible. In some of these scenarios radiography may be diagnostic but most often the appearance is nonspecific and if the clinical situation does not improve within a short time, further investigation may be warranted. In many of these situations ultrasound can be useful.

The ultrasonographic character of bowel loops by simple inspection may reveal normalcy. Personal experience has shown that a uniform distribution of bowel loops that are nondilated and demonstrate peristalsis correlates with no major intraperitoneal process. Even when an infant is not being fed and there is no bowel gas present radiographically, subtle peristaltic movements can be appreciated at ultrasound. In one report of normal controls, it was found that there were a minimum of 10 contractions per minute in each quadrant of the abdomen.[24] Alternatively, lack of peristalsis is nonspecific and can be due to multiple causes.

Malrotation
Malrotation is discussed in the article by Cohen and colleagues elsewhere in this issue. If there is no "swirl" sign of the mesenteric vessels to indicate a volvulus, malrotation still may be present. If an infant is not transportable for a contrast upper GI examination, identifying the transverse duodenum passing posterior to the SMA confirms proper retroperitoneal positioning. With the permission of the physician caring for the baby, a small amount of water may be administered through a nasogastric tube and followed into the duodenum and across the midline to a normal ligament of Treitz, thus excluding this abnormality.

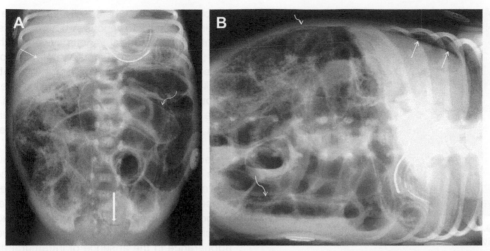

Fig. 17. NEC. (*A*) Supine radiograph shows all of the classic radiographic findings of NEC, with portal venous gas (*thin straight arrow*), intramural gas (*broad arrow*), and extraluminal gas (*curved arrow*) all apparent. (*B*) On the decubitus view, the free air is better seen projecting adjacent to the liver (*straight arrows*) with intramural air again apparent (*curved arrows*).

Necrotizing enterocolitis

NEC is an inflammatory process of uncertain etiology that affects primarily premature infants. The causative factors are probably multiple, including hypoxia, hypotension, infection, an immature intestinal tract with diminished immune response, and inflammatory mediators. The intestinal mucosa becomes involved in the inflammatory process allowing bacterial penetration into the bowel wall with the subsequent development of intramural air and subsequent portal venous air.[26] The clinical symptoms include bowel distension, increased gastric aspirates, bloody stools, temperature instability, and thrombocytopenia.[27] NEC occurs less frequently in full term infants

and is usually due to a specific cause, such as maternal prenatal cocaine use, congenital heart disease or asphyxia, or after gastroschisis repair.[28] Distal ileum and proximal colon are the bowel segments most frequently involved.

A clinical classification of the severity of the disease has been developed by Bell and coworkers and is used in many NICUs. According to this classification, stage I is suspected enterocolitis, stage II is definite enterocolitis, and stage III is severe entercolitis.[29] Once NEC is suspected, clinical management is initiated, including discontinuing feedings, starting antibiotics, and supportive measures. Serial radiographic images are obtained anywhere from every 6 hours to every

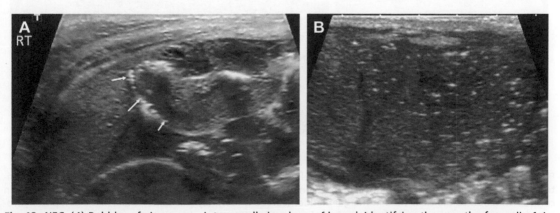

Fig. 18. NEC. (*A*) Bubbles of air are seen intramurally in a loop of bowel. Identifying them on the far wall of the bowel loop (*arrows*) helps to distinguish it from intraluminal air. (*B*) Transverse sonogram of the liver shows portal venous gas as scattered echogenic foci, seen here more throughout the left lobe of the liver than the right.

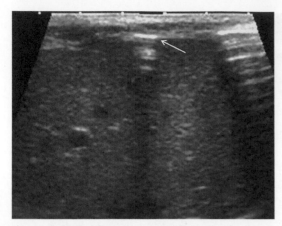

Fig. 19. NEC and free air. Free air (*arrow*) is best seen over liver with a comet tail artifact, where it can be distinguished easily from bowel gas.

12 hours depending on the status of the infant and the local protocol. The films may include only a supine abdomen or an additional horizontal beam image, such as a left lateral decubitus view.

The radiographic findings have been well described in the literature and well summarized by Buonomo.[30] The most common early radiographic pattern is diffuse bowel distension, which can be a nonspecific finding. The development of distended bowel loops that are elongated in configuration, separation of bowel loops, or asymmetric dilatation are somewhat more worrisome for the diagnosis of NEC. A pattern with a fixed dilated loops, as first described by Wexler,[31] is a stronger indication. The diagnosis becomes definite with the appearance of intramural air or portal venous air. This reflects disruption of bowel integrity where air dissects submucosally and appears

bubbly or cystic or subserosally and is more linear. It then can pass into venous structures and subsequently into the portal venous system within the liver (**Fig. 17**). It is documented that ultrasound is more sensitive than plain radiography for detecting small amounts of air within bowel wall or the portal venous system. Intramural air presents as punctuate densities best seen on the dependent wall of a bowel loop or completely circumferential (**Fig. 18**A).

Care must be taken to distinguish intramural air from intraluminal air. It has been reported that bowel wall may become initially thickened and subsequently thin in the presence of necrosis associated with NEC.[25,34,35] Kim and colleagues[34] described two patterns of abnormal bowel wall appearance in the absence of intramural air. The first was a pattern of echogenic dots in the bowel wall and the other was dense granular echogenicities in the bowel wall. The exact nature of the echogenicities are uncertain but Kim and colleagues did identify their disappearance as the disease resolved. Microbubbles of air flowing in the portal vein have an appearance of "fish swimming up stream." Within the liver itself, the air may be scattered diffusely or be seen trapped in smaller veins (**Fig. 18**B).[32,36,37]

Free intraperitoneal air from bowel perforation is felt to be the only finding absolutely requiring surgical intervention. This finding is usually made on a plain radiographic image, sometimes in the supine position but more definitely in a horizontal beam decubitus or cross table lateral view. As with portal venous or intramural air, ultrasound is more sensitive in detecting small amounts of free air, possibly prompting earlier surgical intervention (**Fig. 19**).[25] By ultrasound, free air is most easily

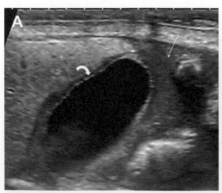
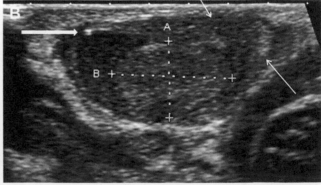

Fig. 20. NEC and bowel perforation. (A) With bowel perforation, echogenic material can be seen within the peritoneum secondary to the development of purulent reaction or bowel contents. It is seen (*straight arrow*) in contradistinction to the clear fluid in the gallbladder (*curved arrow*). (B) This same infant had a complex hydrocele (*thin arrows*) with a single bubble of air from perforation (*broad arrow*) due to the patent processus vaginalis connecting the peritoneal cavity to the scrotum. Cursors (+) connected by dots outline the length (B) and width (A) of the testis.

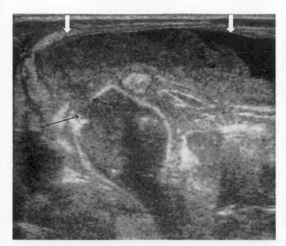

Fig. 21. NEC and bowel perforation. The site of bowel perforation through thin walls is seen (*black arrows*) leading into an adjacent abscess (*broad arrows*).

demonstrated when it is outlined by a solid organ, such as liver or spleen, and remote from air-filled bowel loops.

All of these findings of abnormal air are recorded in the literature. Where ultrasound may be of more benefit is in situations where the neonate is not improving but does not have the classic radiographic findings to determine the status of bowel and peritoneal contents in any detail. One such difficult situation is the radiographic gasless abdomen. Without the presence of gas within bowel lumen, no bowel characteristics can be determined and even the finding of perforation cannot be recognized. In these circumstances, ultrasound can be a critical modality in clinical assessment. One basic

evaluation is for the presence of ascites. Clear fluid is felt to be benign and can be due to multiple causes. Echogenic free fluid could represent blood or purulent material, but in the clinical setting of NEC, bowel perforation with bowel contents or purulent material in the peritoneum may be presumed (**Fig. 20**).[33] In some institutions, this finding alone warrants surgical intervention.[30] The site of perforation usually is not apparent but rarely may demonstrated as a thin intestinal wall with a focal discontinuity (**Fig. 21**).

Doppler assessment may prove a more specific technique than other modalities for evaluating bowel status. Doppler at times, however, can be difficult in the presence of bowel gas, particularly is there is considerable bowel distension where the loops cannot easily be compressed to displace some of the air. If a patient is on an oscillating ventilator, there often is too much vibration from the machine transmitted to the baby causing artifacts with Doppler interrogation.

Increased flow velocities in the celiac axis and SMA have been reported to occur in NEC.[38] This does not help in identifying any specifics as to the status of individual loops or segments of bowel. More recently it has been demonstrated that assessment of bowel viability by color Doppler ultrasound is more sensitive than other modalities.[13,25,35] Faingold found that free air on radiographs was only 40% sensitive for NEC whereas absence of flow to bowel wall was 100% sensitive. Their measurement for normal bowel wall thickness was 1.1 to 2.6 mm. In normal bowel wall they found that color Doppler signal ranged from 1 to 9 dots per square centimeter. Other features in their series are similar to the author's experience,

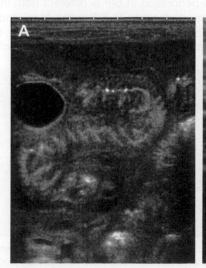
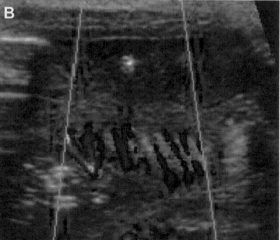

Fig. 22. NEC and bowel hyperemia. (*A*) Transverse sonogram shows a zigzag appearance of the valvulae conniventes indicating edema and hyperemia. (*B*) Increased color Doppler flow confirms hyperemia.

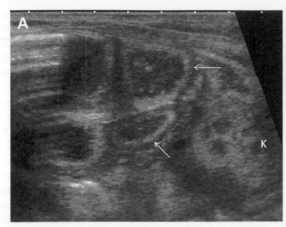
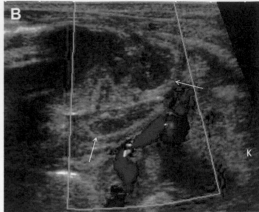

Fig. 23. NEC and bowel necrosis. (*A*) Bowel loops become thickened as they become necrotic, as shown in this transverse sonogram (K, kidney). (*B*) Color Doppler image shows blood flow in the mesentery adjacent to the bowel loops but with no flow to the wall. Subsequently necrotic bowel wall will become thinner and eventually may perforate, as seen in **Fig. 21**.

namely that early on in NEC there may be hyperemia producing increased Doppler flow. This can appear as circumferential flow around the entire bowel loop or color flow along the course of valvulae conniventes (**Fig. 22**).

As bowel wall starts to become ischemic it becomes thickened with decreased blood flow (**Fig. 23**). Vessels may be seen extending to bowel loops but with no flow perfusing the bowel wall itself. This could represent an attempt to reperfuse necrotic bowel, but this could only be documented by serial imaging of the same loop, which is not practical in the usual clinical setting. With further ischemia and necrosis, the bowel wall may become thin before perforation (see **Fig. 21**). Normal loops may be seen adjacent to abnormal loops (**Fig. 24**).

One of the most common complications of NEC is bowel stricture, most commonly in the colon, occurring in 10% to 20% of those who recover.[30] The usual clinical presentation is increased bowel distension but with no other worrisome symptoms. If there has been a diverting ileostomy because of perforation, the stricture may be detected on contrast enema before reanastomosis. For the most part this is diagnosed by contrast enema or antegrade small bowel series. It has been reported that the strictures can be identified by ultrasound, where one study found 19 of 21 strictures in 15 patients.[13] The two strictures missed were in patients with multiple strictures. Because surgeons want to document the distensibility of the bowel, enema is most likely still to be the desired modality of evaluation rather than ultrasound.

Spontaneous intestinal perforation versus necrotizing enterocolitis

Spontaneous intestinal perforation (SIP) is an entity distinct from NEC first recognized more

than 20 years ago[39] and seen in ELBW infants. Risk factors include the administration of indomethacin and steroids, or a combination of the two, during the first week of life.[40–42] Other comorbidities include ventilation, use of pressors, and patent ductus arteriosus. As reported by most investigators, these infants overall are smaller than those with NEC and the perforation occurs at an earlier age, a median of 7 days of life versus 15 days.[41] The clinical presentation in SIP frequently differs from NEC in that infants present with a distended abdomen that is often gasless on plain film radiography. There is a lower incidence of intramural air or portal venous air, and the abdomen develops a bluish discoloration. The bowel perforation usually occurs in the distal ileum within a day of onset of symptoms. The histology of the perforation in SIP is different from in NEC with the perforation in SIP being focal and with no surrounding inflammatory reaction. Some reports have indicated an increase in *Candida* or

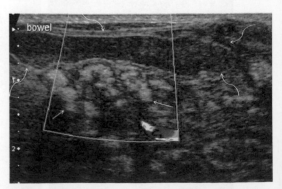

Fig. 24. NEC. Normal decompressed bowel loops are visible with normal color flow (*straight arrows*) with an adjacent fixed, elongated, dilated loop with no peristalsis and no color Doppler flow (*curved arrows*).

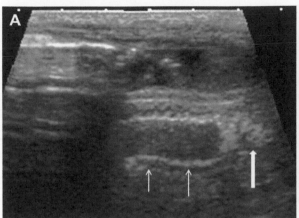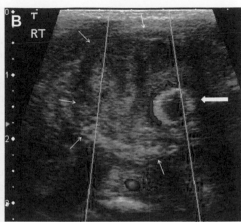

Fig. 25. SIP. This infant did well initially after SIP and then began to deteriorate. (*A*) Longitudinal sonogram shows a fixed dilated loop shown (*straight arrows*) returning to normal caliber (*broad arrow*). (*B*) Transverse sonogram shows the fixed loop is thickened with Doppler flow around it, but not within the bowel wall (*broad arrow*), and with a large surrounding phlegmon (*straight arrows*). At surgery the abnormal loop was the site of the perforation.

Staphylococcus epidermidis infection at the time of surgery in infants with SIP; it is not known whether this is causative or comorbid (**Fig. 25**).[40] The surgical approach may include peritoneal drainage (which often occurs at the bedside due to the unstable status of the infant) or laparotomy with bowel resection.[43,44]

The role of ultrasound in NEC has been described previously. At this time the role of ultrasound in SIP is in detecting complications, such as abscess or subsequent bowel necrosis. If there is prompt recognition by a clinician of the developing symptoms that occur before SIP, ultrasound using Doppler and the other criteria may help in determining bowel status and viability.

SUMMARY

Unlike the abdominal solid organs, the GI tract is more difficult to examine consistently by ultrasound and the evaluation is more user dependent. It can be time consuming and require a great deal of experience to feel comfortable in its evaluation. Using sugar water, Pedialyte, or even breast milk or formula as a contrast agent, mucosal or mural gastric abnormalities can be visualized, gastric outlet obstruction can be examined, and the duodenum can be outlined from pylorus to ligament of Treitz. This requires involvement by a physician in many examinations, as findings are often more apparent during real-time evaluation than on static images.

Although plain radiographs and fluoroscopic studies are often thought of first for GI diseases, ultrasound can provide crucial information in the management of abdominal medical and surgical conditions in infants. For ill infants and those with a gasless abdomen, ultrasound may provide more information than other modalities, and may obviate the need for other examinations. This approach is in keeping with the principal of a ALARA (As Low As Reasonable Achievable), and the goals of the Image Gently campaign that promotes minimization of pediatric radiation exposure when at all possible.[45] Although safe and noninvasive, performing an abdominal ultrasound examination on a VLBW infant or especially an ELBW infant can be stressful to the baby, so close collaboration of the radiologist with the neonatologist and nurses caring for patients is essential.

ACKNOWLEDGMENTS

I am grateful to Michael T. Wallach, MD, for contributing several images and for, by example, challenging me to constantly improve my ultrasound skills.

REFERENCES

1. Teele RL, Share JC. Gastroduodenal ultrasonography. In: Teele RL, Share JC, editors. Ultrasonography of infants and children. Philadelphia: Saunders; 1991. p. 359.
2. Argyropoulou MI, Hadjigeorgi CG, Kiortsis DN. Antro-pyloric canal values from early prematurity to full term gestational age; an ultrasound study. Pediatr Radiol 1998;28(12):933–6.
3. Stringer DA, Daneman A, Brunelle F. Sonography of the normal and abnormal stomach (excluding

hypertrophic pyloric stenosis) in children. J Ultrasound Med 1986;5(4):183–8.

4. McAlister WH, Katz ME, Perlman JM. Sonography of focal foveolar hyperplasia causing gastric obstruction in an infant. Pediatr Radiol 1988;18:79–80.

5. Babyn P, Peled N, Manson D. Radiologic features of gastric outlet obstruction after long term prostaglandin administration. Pediatr Radiol 1995;25(1):41–3.

6. Orzech N, Navarro OM, Langer JC, et al. Is ultrasonography a good screening test for intestinal malrotation? J Pediatr Surg 2006;41(5):1005–9.

7. Yousefzadeh D. The position of the duodenojejunal junction: the wrong horse to bet on in diagnosing or excluding malrotation. Pediatr Radiol 2009; 39(Suppl 2):S172–7.

8. Gomes H, Menanteau B. Gastroesophageal reflux: comparative study between sonography and pH monitoring. Pediatr Radiol 1991;21:168–74.

9. Westra SJ, Wolf BH, Staalman CR. Ultrasound diagnosis of gastroesophageal reflux and hiatal hernia in infants and young children. J Clin Ultrasound 1990; 18(6):477–85.

10. Gomes H, Lallemand A, Lallemand P. Ultrasound of the gastroesophageal junction. Pediatr Radiol 1993; 23(2):94–9.

11. Hernanz-Schulman M. Imaging of neonatal gastrointestinal obstruction. Radiol Clin North Am 1999; 37(6):1163–86.

12. Barnewolt C. Congenital abnormalities of the gastrointestinal tract. Semin Roentgenol 2004;39(2):263–81.

13. Couture A. Bowel obstruction in neonates and children. In: Baert AL, Knauth M, Sartor K, editors. Gastrointestinal tract sonography in fetuses and children. Berlin: Springer; 2008. p. 136, 189, 199–207.

14. Schlesinger AE. Duodenum: congenital anomalies. In: Slovis TL, editor. 11th edition, Caffey's pediatric diagnostic imaging, vol. 2. Philadelphia: Mosby Elsevier; 2008. p. 2109–14.

15. Siegel M. Gastrointestinal tract. In: Pediatric sonography. 3rd edition. Philadelphia: Lippincott Williams & Wilkins; 2002. p. 349.

16. Segal SR, Sherman NH, Rosenberg HK, et al. Ultrasonographic features of gastrointestinal duplications. J Ultrasound Med 1994;13(11):863–70.

17. Neal MR, Seibert JJ, Vanderzahn T, et al. Neonatal ultrasonography to distinguish between meconium ileus and ileal atresia. J Ultrasound Med 1997;16:263–6.

18. Finkel LI, Slovis TL. Meconium peritonitis, intraperitoneal calcifications and cystic fibrosis. Pediatr Radiol 1982;12:92–3.

19. Foster MA, Nyberg DA, Mahony BS, et al. Meconium peritonitis: prenatal sonographic findings and their clinical significance. Radiology 1987; 165:661–5.

20. Dirkes K, Cromblehome TM, Craigo SD, et al. The natural history of meconium peritonitis diagnosed in utero. J Pediatr Surg 1995;30:979–82.

21. Swischuk LE. Alimentary tract. In: Imaging of the newborn, infant, and young child. 5th edition. Philadelphia: Lippincott Williams & Wilkins; 2004. p. 464.

22. Han TII, Kim I-O, Kim WS. Imperforate anus: US determination of the type with infracoccygeal approach. Radiology 2003;228:226–9.

23. Dietrich RB, Rogh GM. Pediatric body. In: Stark DD, Bradley WG, editors, Magnetic resonance imaging, vol. 1. St. Louis (MO): Mosby; 1999. p. 663.

24. Faingold R, Daneman A, Tomlinson G, et al. Necrotizing enterocolitis: assessment of bowel viability with color Doppler US. Radiology 2005;235(2):587–94.

25. Silva CT, Daneman A, Navarro OM. Correlation of sonographic findings and outcome in necrotizing enterocolitis. Pediatr Radiol 2007;37(3):274–82.

26. Vieten D, Corfield A, Carroll D. Impaired mucosal regeneration in neonatal necrotizing enterocolitis. Pediatr Surg Int 2005;21(3):153–60.

27. Bertino E, Giuliani F, Prandi G, et al. Necrotizing enterocolitis: risk factor analysis and role of gastric residuals in very low birth weight infants. J Pediatr Gastroenterol Nutr 2009;48(4):437–42.

28. Ostlie DJ, Spilde TL, St Peter SD, et al. Necrotizing enterocolitis in full term infants. J Pediatr Surg 2004;38(7):1039–42.

29. Bell MJ, Ternberg JL, Feigin RD, et al. Neonatal necrotizing enterocolitis. Therapeutic decisions based upon clinical staging. Ann Surg 1978; 187(1):1–7.

30. Buonomo C. The radiology of necrotizing enterocolitis. Radiol Clin North Am 1999;37(6):1187–98.

31. Wexler H. The persistent loop sign in neonatal necrotizing enterocolitis: a new indication for surgical intervention? Radiology 1978;126:201–14.

32. Lindley S, Mollitt DL, Seibert JJ, et al. Portal vein ultrasonography in the early diagnosis of necrotizing enterocolitis. J Pediatr Surg 1986;21(6):530–2.

33. Miller SF, Seibert JJ, Kinder DL, et al. Use of ultrasound in the detection of occult bowel perforation in neonates. J Ultrasound Med 1993;12(9):531–5.

34. Kim WY, Kim WS, Kim IO, et al. Sonographic evaluation of neonates with early-stage necrotizing enterocolitis. Pediatr Radiol 2005;35(11):1056–61.

35. Epelman M, Daneman A, Navarro OM. Necrotizing enterocolitis: review of state-of-the-art imaging findings with pathologic correlation. Radiographics 2007;27:285–305.

36. Goske MJ, Goldblum JR, Applegate KE, et al. The "circle sign": a new sonographic sign of pneumatosis intestinalis—clinical, pathologic and experimental findings. Pediatr Radiol 1999;29:530–5.

37. Merritt CR, Goldsmith JP, Sharp MJ. Sonographic detection of portal venous gas in infants with necrotizing enterocolitis. AJR Am J Roentgenol 1984; 143(5):1059–62.

38. Deeg DH, Rupprecht T, Schmid E. Doppler sonographic detection of increased flow velocities in

the celiac trunk and superior mesenteric artery in infants with necrotizing enterocolitis. Pediatr Radiol 1993;23:578.

39. Aschner JJ, Deluga KS, Metlay LA, et al. Spontaneous focal gastrointestinal perforation in very low birth weight infants. J Pediatr 1988;113:364–7.

40. Gordon PV, Attridge JT. Understanding clinical literature relevant to spontaneous intestinal perforations. Am J Perinatol 2009;26(4):309–16.

41. Attridge JT, Clark C, Walker MW. New insights into spontaneous intestinal perforation using a national data set: (1) SIP is associated with early indomethacin exposure. J Perinatol 2006;26:93–9.

42. Stark AR, Carlo WA, Tyson JE, et al. Adverse effects of early dexamethasone treatment in extremely-low-birth-weight infants. N Engl J Med 2001;344(2):95–101.

43. Hunter CJ, Chokshi N, Ford HR. Evidence vs. experience in the surgical management of necrotizing entercolitis and focal intestinal perforation. J Perinatol 2008;28(Suppl 1):S14–7.

44. Blakely ML, Lally KP, McDonald S, et al. Postoperative outcomes of extremely low birth-weight infants with necrotizing entercolitis or isolated intestinal perforation. Ann Surg 2005;241(6):984–94.

45. Willis CE, Slovis TL. The ALARA concept in pediatric CR and DR: dose reduction in pediatric radiographic exams—a white paper conference executive summary. Pediatr Radiol 2004;34(Suppl 3):S162–4.

The Vomiting Neonate or Young Infant

Harris L. Cohen, MD[a,b,c],*, Elton B. Greene, MD[d],
Thomas P. Boulden, MD[a,b]

KEYWORDS

- Neonatal vomiting • Hypertrophic pyloric stenosis
- Pylorospasm • Ultrasound

This article reviews the clinical concerns and imaging approaches needed to diagnose the cause of vomiting in children in the first months of life.

Imaging approaches to any given problem evolve. This evolution occurs as individuals and groups gain years of experience with specific imaging modalities and as changes take place in the ordering "culture" of a given subspecialty, clinical department, local health delivery system, state, or country. Imaging choices within nations, regions, and hospitals, and among individual practitioners often relate to past training of staff. Such choices include those related to orders and workups by primary clinicians, and, in the case of vomiting, gastroenterologists and surgeons, as well as the imagers of the affected patient group, usually the radiologists.[1] Radiologists, in particular, may be influenced by expert panel reports from their national organizations (eg, the American College of Radiology).[2] Ultrasonologists are affected by guidelines and appropriateness criteria produced by their subspecialty organizations (eg, the American Institute of Ultrasound in Medicine and the Society of Radiologists in Ultrasound). A recent and welcome trend has been the creation of joint guidelines created across subspecialty and specialty organizational lines. There is also a necessity to consider other factors in workups. In the case of pediatric vomiting, such factors include radiation exposure because of

the national concern regarding excessive radiation exposure from imaging workups that use radiation to make diagnoses (eg, plain radiographs, fluoroscopy, and, particularly because of its increasing use in emergency workups, computed tomography).[3] Image Gently is an example of a highly respected educational and advocacy group for patients that seeks to limit excessive diagnostic radiation exposures. Radiologists, clinicians, physicists, and imaging equipment manufacturers, among those who make up its membership and advisory groups, seek controlled radiation exposures in diagnostic workups with the ultimate goal being safer diagnoses.[4] When radiation needs to be used for diagnosis, it should be used. However, use of radiation needs to be prudent, as expressed in the ALARA (as low as reasonably achievable) principle. This has been the authors' goal for decades and ultrasound has been a most helpful tool to this end.[5]

In 2000, the American College of Radiology's expert panel on pediatric imaging began producing appropriateness criteria based on given symptoms. The panel of experts determined best and alternative methods for a workup to diagnose the cause of specific symptoms based on clinical imaging experience and evidence-based literature. In coauthoring information on vomiting in infants up to 3 months of age, the authors chose to sort infants with this problem into three groups: the newborn with bilious vomiting, the child with

[a] Department of Radiology, University of Tennessee Health Science Center, 150 Chandler Building, Memphis, TN 38163, USA
[b] Department of Radiology, LeBonheur Children's Medical Center, 50 North Dunlop, Memphis, TN 38103, USA
[c] Pediatrics and Obstetrics and Gynecology, Memphis, TN, USA
[d] Department of Radiology, University of Tennessee, Methodist University Hospital Program, Memphis, TN, USA
* Corresponding author. 5639 Ashley Square S, Memphis, TN 38120.
E-mail address: hcohenmb@optonline.net

Ultrasound Clin 5 (2010) 97–112
doi:10.1016/j.cult.2009.11.017

intermittent vomiting since birth, and the child with projectile vomiting developing after several weeks of healthy life.[2] This review article uses that division to better review the various considerations for vomiting in the first months of life.

Vomiting is the forceful extrusion of gastric contents. It is never normal in the neonate. It usually occurs because of complete or partial obstruction somewhere along the course of the gastrointestinal (GI) tract between the stomach and cecum.[6] However, the ability to differentiate clinically between vomiting and regurgitation, a common finding in the first 3 months of life, is difficult. The most common cause for vomiting during the first three 3 months of life is gastroesophageal reflux (GER), which is the regurgitation of stomach contents. This "spitting up" is extremely common and, most often, easily recognized as such. At times, such regurgitation may simulate true vomiting. Parents, especially first-time parents, may mistake it for true vomiting. GER simulating vomiting must be considered, but there are a number of other causes to consider. In the first months of life, neonatal sepsis, hypertrophic pyloric stenosis (HPS), and pylorospasm are key possibilities that must be taken into consideration.[2]

Necrotizing enterocolitis is a consideration among premature infants in a neonatal intensive care unit setting. The most frequent cause of medical surgical emergencies and the most common cause for bowel perforation in neonates, necrotizing enterocolitis is of unclear etiology, but is perhaps related to intestinal hypoxia. Clinical findings can include abdominal distention, a common neonatal finding in many without the disease. Vomiting, but more often feeding intolerance, suggests the diagnosis, as do bloody stools. Plain radiograph findings, including persistent abnormal bowel loops, air in bowel wall (pneumatosis intestinalis) (**Fig. 1**), portal venous air or free air (sometimes requiring left side down decubitus radiographs shot cross table), can make the diagnosis.[7] Ultrasound has been used by some to make the diagnosis (see previous issue of *Ultrasound Clinics*). Punctate echogenicities in the liver may suggest portal venous air, a diagnosis more easily made when imaging the echogenicities in flowing portal venous blood. Air can be noted in bowel wall as tiny echogenicities whose position within the bowel wall may be confirmed by transducer pressure.[7–9]

Among the less common causes of vomiting is bowel malrotation with midgut volvulus, a clinically emergent condition. Vomiting, however, may also be caused by malrotation without volvulus. Other less common causes include congenital atresia or stenoses of small bowel, and functional

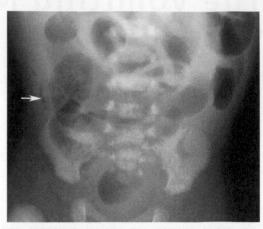

Fig. 1. Air in bowel wall. Anteroposterior abdominal plain radiograph. Radiolucency seen around the bowel lumen (*arrow*) is consistent with bowel wall air, which was seen in this neonatal intensive care unit patient with bowel distention and necrotizing enterocolitis.

obstructions of the small or large bowel, including Hirschsprung disease, small left colon syndrome, and meconium ileus or meconium plug syndrome. Even rarer causes of vomiting of GI origin developing in the first months of life include neonatal appendicitis, intussusception, gastric ulcer disease, and lactobezoars. Vomiting may also be due to extra-GI causes, particularly those affecting the central nervous system. These include subdural collections, drugs or toxic agents, and such medical conditions as kernicterus, metabolic disorders, or causes of renal failure.[2,10–12]

DIAGNOSTIC IMAGING MODALITIES

The first step in the imaging evaluation of the vomiting neonate is the abdominal plain radiograph. This may be aided by an upright or decubitus radiograph for free air, if suspected. Decubitus radiographs are usually performed with left side down to allow radiolucent free air to be seen against the white background of the liver. Key in the analysis of obstruction is the bowel gas pattern. At times an incidental air-filled esophagus may be seen in a child with reflux. Certainly a dilated stomach, but more so, dilated small bowel (especially if there is no more distal bowel gas), may suggest obstruction, especially if seen similarly on a follow-up radiograph. The stomach may be filled with air from crying. The "caterpillar" sign (**Fig. 2**) has been used as the term for a dilated stomach with a somewhat undulating greater and lesser curve due to peristalsis against a relative obstruction, the relatively obstructed pylorus in HPS.[13] Plain radiographs showing definitive small

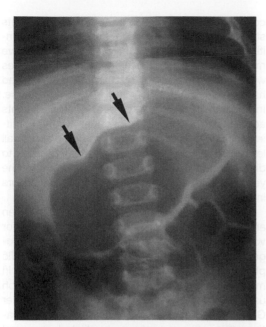

Fig. 2. Caterpillar sign of HPS on plain radiograph. Within the upper abdomen of a 4-week-old infant with HPS is an air-filled structure with undulant borders (*arrows*) consistent with the stomach. The borders, likened to a caterpillar seen walking from above, are due to peristalsis against a relative obstruction, the pylorus.

bowel obstruction may end further imaging workup in a newborn by suggesting the need for surgery for small bowel atresia. However, in many instances, the plain radiograph will reveal no information. Negative plain radiographs in a patient with worrisome clinical findings should certainly not preclude further imaging.[2]

The necessary question to answer in the analysis of the vomiting neonate and infant is whether there is a true mechanical/surgical obstruction. The best methodology to answer that question is to image the stomach and small bowel. Historically, to assess the stomach and small bowel, many radiologists used and still use barium in an upper GI series. Some centers use lower osmolarity contrast agents for extremely ill or very premature infants. The barium or other contrast material is used to evaluate the luminal stomach, the egress of contrast from stomach antrum through the pyloric channel into the duodenum, and then the movement of barium through the duodenum to its fourth portion at the ostensible area of the ligament of Treitz.[2,11,14,15] The normal duodenum begins with the bulb, to the right of the antrum, and then descends inferiorly (sometimes taking an elongated "watch fob" course to the right) as the second portion of the duodenum,

and then courses horizontally to the left, as the third and fourth portions of the duodenum, to the left of the vertebral column and upward normally to the level of the duodenal bulb, suggesting a normal position for the ligament of Treitz and thus no malrotation. The small bowel will continue as jejunum on the left side of the abdomen.

Investigators at least as far back as the early 1980s at the beginnings of readily available real-time ultrasound have used echoless water as a contrast agent that can provide much of the information obtained with barium. It is somewhat operator dependent, but as with good magnetic resonance and computed tomography work, devoted imagers can obtain better images than dilettantes. A "highly operator dependent" examination should be a challenge to learn and perfect rather than a reason to avoid a modality. Fluid-aided ultrasound can be quite successful in real-time imaging of gastric emptying and of GER into the lower esophagus, as well as in diagnosing HPS, its simulator pylorospasm, and various duodenal abnormalities, including midgut volvulus. Using water as an ultrasound contrast agent, one can examine the patient for minutes, assessing stomach and duodenal real-time activity without the fear or consequences of overzealous fluoroscopy and its radiation exposure.[16–18] Incidentally, in recent years, ultrasound work using water or echoless nonabsorbable solutions, such as polyethylene glycol, have advanced ultrasound intraluminal bowel analysis of the jejunum, ileum, and colon.[18] Improvements in fluoroscopic equipment have decreased overall radiation exposures. However, time is still an enemy in fluoroscopy. Well-planned examinations with specific points to discover (and, in the opinion of the authors, aided by nasogastric tube placement if the patient is not drinking well enough to fill the stomach) can keep fluoroscopic times controlled. The upper GI series does provide a more global view of the upper GI tract, whereas only portions of the fluid-filled GI tract can be noted on individual images obtained by ultrasound.[2] Luminal gas limits ultrasound imaging.

WORKUPS AND DIAGNOSTIC CONSIDERATIONS AMONG VOMITING NEONATES

Not all vomiting scenarios in babies in the first months of life are of similar presentation. As stated earlier, a review of three common scenarios can help the reader assess the thought processes and imaging decisions used for diagnosis. The role of ultrasound in these diagnoses will be discussed.

Scenario 1: Bilious Vomiting in the Newborn

Regurgitation of occasional feedings in the first days to months of life is a very common physiologic phenomenon. At times, separating the common GER from a potentially more severe abnormality inducing true vomiting is difficult clinically. The frequency, quality, and quantity of the regurgitated material can provide important clues. Physicians can place the child in the first 3 months of life who has nonbilious vomiting under closer clinical surveillance.[2,19,20] Bilious or "green" vomitus, however, is a matter of urgent medical concern. It is usually the result of sepsis or obstruction and is considered a radiologic emergency because, if it is due to obstruction caused by volvulus of the midgut about the superior mesenteric artery (SMA), bowel fed by that vessel is at risk for infarction. A quick and accurate diagnosis is necessary. Volvulus often occurs when the bowel has rotated improperly and it and its mesentery are not attached normally to the retroperitoneum. Normally, bowel develops embryologically between weeks 6 and 10 of gestation from a single tube into the luminal GI tract that eventually, after a 270° turn about the SMA, is in part made up of a stomach on the left side of the abdomen, a right-sided descending duodenum, a transverse duodenum that crosses from the right abdomen into the left abdomen, and a distal (fourth portion) of the duodenum, which attaches to the ligament of Treitz, within the left abdomen at the same height as the duodenal bulb and superior to the celiac axis, at the duodenojejunal junction. Abnormalities of bowel layout most often develop during the first 90° of rotation, which occurs extracoelomically, within the base of the umbilical cord. During week 10 of gestation, the midgut returns into the abdomen, cranial end first. This return of physiologically normal herniated bowel should be complete by week 12 of gestation. "If the small bowel fails to reenter the abdomen in a normal fashion, or if the distal duodenum fails to attach to the ligament of Treitz, or if the normal broad mesenteric band attaching small bowel from the ligament of Treitz to the ileocecal valve is absent, or if Ladd's bands or other points of abnormal fixation are present, the result may be malrotation with the potential for midgut volvulus and its associated compromise of SMA flow to the bowel."[2] The small bowel distal to a volvulus may therefore infarct in severe cases or become ischemic in less severe cases. Small bowel ischemia may lead to the development of small bowel atresia or stenosis.[2,10,21]

The necessity to treat bilious vomiting as a radiologic emergency because of possible volvulus continues even though only 20% of 45 patients studied by Lilien and colleagues[14] for bilious vomiting in the first 72 hours of life were found to have midgut volvulus. Greater than two thirds of cases were not the result of obstruction, but instead had an idiopathic cause and a transient course. In addition, 11% of their bilious vomiting patients actually had a lower GI tract cause for the vomiting, including meconium plug syndrome and small left colon syndrome. Clinicians must be able to differentiate true bilious (green) vomiting from the yellow colostrum or meconium vomitus that occurs in unusual cases of distal bowel obstruction.

From an imaging perspective, only 44% of Lilien and colleagues' patients who required surgery for volvulus had a definitively positive plain radiograph. The remainder had normal or nonspecific plain radiographs. This is a common finding in midgut volvulus cases. Where the plain radiograph usually fails to show abnormality, both the upper GI series and the fluid-aided ultrasound examination (Fig. 3) can show a dilated proximal duodenum with a beak or twist at the point of obstruction of the proximal small bowel in cases of midgut volvulus.[2,16] In making the imaging diagnosis, only a small amount of fluid or barium should be placed into the stomach for the assessment and diagnosis so as to avoid reflux of the material and potential aspiration. When using ultrasound for the examination, one could possibly use fluid already present in the stomach for the analysis.[2]

Normal bowel rotation can be confirmed by following the barium of an upper GI series or the echoless fluid (water) of a fluid-aided ultrasound (Fig. 4) to the ligament of Treitz. It is harder to see the complete duodenum using ultrasound. However, one can see the fourth portion of the duodenum filled with fluid just posterior to the stomach and this can enable assessment of the height in relationship to the duodenal bulb. Ultrasound with water (hydrosonography) or the upper GI series with barium can enable imaging of the layout of the duodenum and prove normal bowel rotation or note abnormal or nonrotation of bowel, including jejunum that fills predominantly on the right side of the abdomen (Fig. 5). It is true, however, that even in the best of hands, deciding what is normal bowel rotation even by the upper GI series may prove difficult. Opinions have changed regarding what is normal based in part on reexamined upper GI series' after positive operative findings. Radiologists are now stricter about having the fourth portion of duodenum positioned at a height similar to that of the duodenal bulb.[2,22]

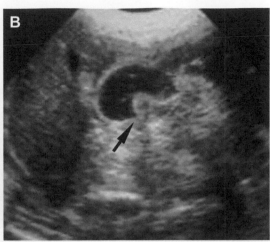

Fig. 3. Midgut volvulus. (*A*) Upper GI series. The contrast-filled descending duodenum (D) is dilated to a point of relative narrowing where it twists (*arrow*) and travels inferiorly rather than crossing to the right side of the abdomen and up toward the ligament of Treitz, as would occur normally. The dilatation was due to the gut being relatively obstructed at a point where slightly more distal bowel twisted about the SMA (not able to be seen) in this case of midgut volvulus in a 1-day-old with bilious vomiting. (*B*) Ultrasound. A fluid-filled descending duodenum ends in a beaked end (*arrow*), also due to a twist in the gut just distal to it in another case of midgut volvulus in a newborn with bilious vomiting.

Ultrasound has also been used to suggest possible bowel malrotation when an abnormal relationship between aorta and inferior vena cava in relation to the position of the SMA and superior mesenteric vein (SMV) are noted. The SMA, with its surrounding echogenic rim (**Fig. 6**), should be

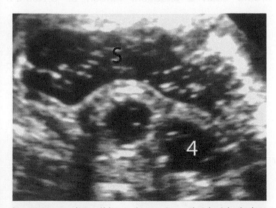

Fig. 4. Normal small bowel rotation. Fluid-aided ultrasound. Transverse plane. Fluid and milk debris are seen in the stomach (S). Posterior to it but at the same level is fluid in the third and fourth (4) portions of the duodenum that were followed from antrum to this point posterior to the stomach and at the same height as the duodenal bulb (not shown). Findings suggest normal rotation with normal position of the ligament of Treitz. (*From* Blumer S, Zucconi W, Cohen HL, et al. The vomiting neonate: a review of the ACR appropriateness criteria and ultrasound's role in the workup of such patients. Ultrasound Q 2004;20:81; with permission.)

seen in front of the aorta and to the left of the SMV, which is normally found anterior to the inferior vena cava. Weinberger and colleagues[23] reported four of four cases with reversal of the normal relationship (ie, the SMV was seen to the left of the SMA and anterior to the aorta) had bowel malrotation (**Fig. 7**). One in four of their cases in which SMV and SMA were situated in front of each other in an anterior-to-posterior position, rather than a side-to-side position, also had malrotation. Ultrasound can usually quickly assess the SMA and its position by noting its echogenic rim or arterial pulsation or Doppler arterial spectral pattern.

Less common reported causes of bilious vomiting include supradiaphragmatic herniation of the stomach (eg, hiatal hernias) (**Fig. 8**) and unusual cases of gastric volvulus.[2,24]

Scenario 2: Intermittent Vomiting that has Occurred Since Birth

GER is the most common cause of what is seen by the parents as intermittent vomiting.[2] At least some GER can be elicited in almost all children less than 3 months old. It is thought to occur so commonly in neonates because of an age-related "immaturity" of the lower esophageal sphincter. GER, however, is not the only cause of intermittent vomiting occurring since birth in neonates. Other causes one must consider range from the relatively common pylorospasm to the less common gastric volvulus or gastric ulcers.[2,17,25,26]

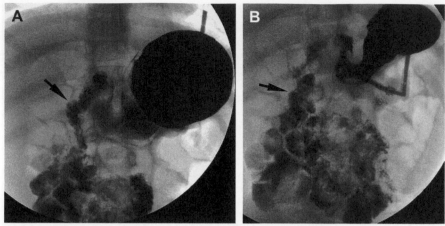

Fig. 5. Small bowel malrotation without volvulus. Upper GI series. (A) Contrast placed through a gastrostomy tube was noted to extend from stomach to descending duodenum on the right side of the abdomen. The duodenum (arrow) does not cross over to the left side of the abdomen and rise to the level of the duodenal bulb, as would be expected for the normal position of the ligament of Treitz. Rather, the duodenum remains on the right side continuing inferiorly. (B) The duodenum (arrow) and jejunum run predominantly on the right rather than the left side of the abdomen. There was no volvulus of small bowel. The images, however, indicate that the patient's small bowel is malrotated (sometimes called dysrotated or nonrotated) in relationship to the SMA (which is not imaged). Barium examinations give a more global view of the duodenal layout than does ultrasound.

A 1991 article by O'Keefe and colleagues[27] reviewed the cases of 145 infants who presented with intermittent vomiting. Of those 145 patients, 43 (30%) had GER as the cause while 40 cases (27.5%) were due to HPS, a diagnosis more often associated with projectile vomiting after weeks of normal life. Nineteen percent of cases (n = 27) were thought to be the result of overfeeding. A neonate with a voracious appetite may overfill his or her stomach. A parent who does not pay attention to a feed and intermittent burping may also create such a situation. Fifteen of O'Keefe's

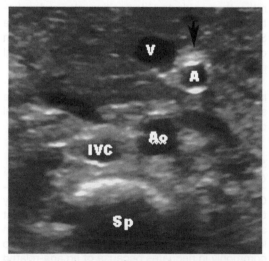

Fig. 6. Normal SMA. Ultrasound. Transverse plane. The normal SMA (A) has an echogenic rim (arrow). No echogenic rim surrounds the SMV (V). There is a normal SMA/SMV relationship. The SMA is to the left of the right-sided SMV. The SMA is essentially anterior to the aorta (Ao), while the SMV is anterior to the inferior vena cava (IVC). Sp, spine.

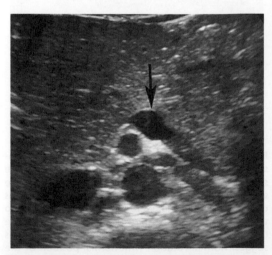

Fig. 7. Abnormal SMA/SMV relationship. Ultrasound. Transverse plane. The SMV (arrow) is seen to the left of the SMA and its echogenic wall. This abnormal relationship has been associated with small bowel malrotation, which this patient had.

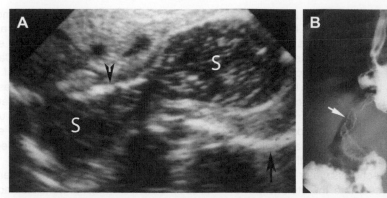

Fig. 8. Hiatal hernia. (*A*) Ultrasound. Fluid- and debris-filled stomach (*S*) is seen on both sides of midline. Portion of stomach to the reader's right (*left S*) is seen anterior and therefore below the diaphragm (*arrow*) while portion of the stomach on the reader's left (*right S*) is posterior to the diaphragm (*arrowhead*), suggesting that that portion is superior to the diaphragm and therefore is an intrathoracic hernia, which proved to be a hiatal hernia. (*B*) Upper GI series. A barium contrast examination proves the stomach (*S*) at the time of the examination to be completely superior to the diaphragm. The straight descent of the duodenum (*arrow*) without a horizontal turn suggests malrotation/nonrotation of the small bowel (*From* Blumer S, Zucconi W, Cohen HL, et al. The vomiting neonate: a review of the ACR appropriateness criteria and ultrasound's role in the workup of such patients. Ultrasound Q 2004;20:81; with permission.)

patients had pylorospasm, 14 had milk allergy, and 1 had gastroenteritis as the eventually discovered cause of intermittent vomiting.

The current gold standard test in the diagnostic workup for GER is extended pH probe monitoring. However, there are concerns and controversies with regard to its usage. It is a somewhat invasive and technically demanding examination, particularly for a finding that is said to occur physiologically at 40 refluxes in 24 hours or 1.6 refluxes per hour.[28] It is limited in assessing short-term or neutral pH refluxes. The pH monitoring may prove negative yet the patient may still have the symptoms of GER disease, which include regurgitation, choking, irritability, and failure to thrive. In any case, this concern is greater for an older child than for the infant 3 months old or younger. The Tuttle test and esophageal motility studies are said to be unreliable in young children. Imaging studies are performed to prove reflux of gastric contents into the esophagus. But more often, their key importance is in proving that there is no more distal anatomic obstruction as the cause. Knowledge regarding emptying of the stomach is key as is knowledge of whether material from the stomach refluxed into the esophagus. Important findings to note with regard to esophageal studies, however, are the degree of reflux based on the number of events for a given time, the height of the refluxing column, the quality of the esophageal mucosa, and evidence of aspiration into the lungs.[2,28]

Imaging examinations can denote GER to a variable degree. Plain radiographs do not play a role in

the diagnosis of GER. In one study, Swischuk and colleagues[29] noted an air-filled esophagus of at least 1 cm in diameter on chest radiograph, which they termed megaesophagus, in 16 chronic vomiters who proved to have GER or esophageal obstruction. Many pediatric radiologists use a portion of their fluoroscopy time assessing patients for GER. The examination, ideally, can diagnose GER via swallowed or nasogastric tube–placed barium. The authors use an amount of barium equivalent to at least one half of the patient's typical feed, preferring to place it into the stomach via an 8F-catheter 15-in nasogastric tube, especially if the patient does not drink at a reasonable pace and the parents approve. This is to decrease radiation exposure times, to challenge the antropyloric area with a large feed, and to readily note whether there is any malrotation or other abnormality of the stomach or the duodenum as the cause of reflux. Ideally, the barium study would separate infants who have significant reflux up to the level of the clavicles from those who have no reflux or reflux to a minor extent into the distal esophagus. However, the conventional barium examination is said to be only 43% sensitive for reflux disease.[28] Despite this, the upper GI series has been reported as more sensitive, but less specific, for this than the pH probe examination.[11]

Nuclear medicine (nuclear meal) scintigraphy can be used to image for reflux over time at an overall total radiation dose lower than that of the upper GI series. However, the protocols and interpretation criteria of this nuclear medicine examination, especially in a child less than 3 months old, are not standardized. Many agree that, because of this and the insensitivity of the nuclear medicine meal to detect aspiration, its use should be limited to children older than 3 months with failure to thrive who have been proven to be without an anatomic obstruction as the cause of regurgitation or reflux.[2,11,30,31]

Ultrasound can be used to diagnose reflux by observing water placed into the stomach refluxing into the distal esophagus. The authors usually place about 60 mL of echoless water or Pedialyte fluid (half of a 4-oz feed) into the stomach. The distal esophagus and stomach are studied both in a transverse plane at the level of the diaphragm and its esophageal hiatus and in a longitudinal plane through the midline, and angled slightly leftward, resulting in an image of the distal esophagus anterior to the aorta. The left lobe of the liver is often used as a window in this midline longitudinal maneuver. The nasogastric tube is removed before analysis to avoid reflux resulting from a tube crossing the gastroesophageal junction. Reflux is noted by echoless fluid rising from the stomach into the distal esophagus (**Fig. 9**).[2,17,32,33]

Riccabona and colleagues[34] found ultrasound to be 100% sensitive and 87.5% specific in diagnosing GER. Cohen and colleagues[17] found ultrasound to be successful in diagnosing 48 true-positive and 6 true-negative cases of GER with only 1 false negative. Although ultrasound

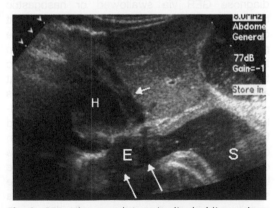

Fig. 9. GER. Ultrasound. Longitudinal oblique plane. The patient's head is toward the reader's left. Relatively echoless fluid, seen in the stomach (S), had been placed there by a nasogastric tube. The esophagus was empty. During the examination, fluid refluxed (*long arrows*) into the esophagus (E). That fluid, seen as relatively echoless material within the esophagus, rose above the diaphragm (*short arrow*). H, heart. (*From* Blumer S, Zucconi W, Cohen HL, et al. The vomiting neonate: a review of the ACR appropriateness criteria and ultrasound's role in the workup of such patients. Ultrasound Q 2004;20:84; with permission.)

can provide functional as well as morphologic information,[33,34] it does not allow analysis of mucosa and certainly cannot see the esophagus higher than its lower third. McCauley and colleagues[35] discussed the concept of prominent esophageal width at the GE junction as evidence of more significant reflux using the upper GI series. We make a similar assumption with ultrasound. Hence, the more dilated the distal esophagus appears at reflux, the more likely the degree of reflux is significant.

Color Doppler ultrasound has been used to assess motion of material from stomach into the esophagus. Hirsch and colleagues,[36] in comparing its use to pH probe testing, found a greater sensitivity at 98% compared with 84% but a poor negative predictive rate—as low as 33%. Jang and colleagues[37] noted 94% agreement between pH testing and ultrasound with color Doppler for GER.[28]

Gastric ulcers are traditionally diagnosed by the upper GI series or endoscopy. They are not a usual imaging finding in the first 3 months of life. Hayden and colleagues[26] used ultrasound to diagnose what were confirmed to be gastric ulcers in seven infants; six had the complaint of chronic vomiting and one had syncope with "coffee ground vomitus." Ultrasound demonstrated mucosal thickening of more than 4 mm with a sharp delineation of the normal and abnormal gastric wall regions. Each affected patient also showed delayed gastric emptying.[18,26,38]

Chronic gastric volvulus is not as uncommon as once believed. In the infant and neonate, the primary presentation is recurrent vomiting.[2] There are no characteristic plain radiograph findings. An upper GI may demonstrate gastric volvulus as a stomach with an elevated greater curvature, the greater curve of the stomach crossing the esophagus, a downward presenting pylorus, two different stomach air–fluid levels, or a more caudal than typical gastric fundal position.[39] Patients with gastric volvulus certainly may reflux. They may have recurrent vomiting associated with clinical complaints of abrupt episodic cyanosis and apnea, anorexia, or pneumonia.[2,40] Certainly typical and more complex hiatal hernias seen on ultrasound as the stomach, or a portion of it, in a position higher than the diaphragm can similarly be responsible for reflux or vomiting (see **Fig. 8**).[2]

Two additional differential considerations for intermittent vomiting since birth include HPS and pylorospasm (discussed in detail in the next scenario because they more typically present as projectile vomiting, usually developing after several weeks of life without any vomiting).

Scenario 3: Projectile Vomiting Developing after Several Weeks in a Previously Healthy Child

Nonbilious projectile vomiting developing after several weeks of normal life has a different differential diagnosis than the already discussed scenarios. The key considerations include GER (already discussed) and pylorospasm with the primary concern being HPS. Historical and clinical information helps the analysis. Imaging, particularly ultrasound, makes the diagnosis. The following discussion will concentrate on HPS and pylorospasm.

Hypertrophic pyloric stenosis

HPS most typically presents after 3 weeks and not usually beyond 6 weeks of age. Because of the current ease of diagnosis using ultrasound, attempts at making the diagnosis at an earlier age are becoming more common. Goske and Schlesinger[41] state that the diagnosis is usually made between 3 weeks and 3 months and indicate that cases can be discovered even in the first weeks of life. The authors have seen a few in the first weeks of life, often with a smaller ultrasound measurement than one would have expected at a later age, but have not seen a case beyond 9 weeks of age.

HPS is more common in first-born males. Boys are affected about four times as often as girls. Five to seven percent of patients have a positive family history. The positive family history, for unknown reasons, is more often on the mother's side, typically involving her male relatives, by a ratio of 4:1. There is an increase in likelihood of HPS developing in the twin and triplet siblings of an affected patient.[5,41,42] HPS has been reported to occur at 2 to 5 cases per 1000 births among whites, with the incidence varying in different geographic areas. It is less common in India and within black and Asian populations, with a frequency approximately one third to one fifth that of the white population.[5,43]

The etiology of HPS is unknown. Besides the obvious linkage to an inherited, probably genetic cause, numerous other factors have been linked to its causation. One theory suggests that abnormal innervation of the muscular layer of the pylorus (either because of decreased ganglion cells and neurofibrils in the pylorus or immaturity of the ganglion cells in the pyloric region) leads to failed muscle relaxation, increased synthesis of growth factors, and subsequent hypertrophy and hyperplasia of the pylorus.[5,44] Another theory has implicated hypergastrinemia and hyperacidity proposing that an inherited increase in parietal

cells in the affected region initiates a cycle of increased acid production, repeated pyloric contraction, and delayed gastric emptying.[5,45] Supporting this is the fact that HPS is said to develop only after the initiation of feedings and is found in the presence of high postprandial gastrin levels and markedly increased gastric acid secretion. Pentagastric infusion has been used to induce HPS in puppies.[5,46]

Whatever the cause of HPS, spasm and edema of the pyloric mucosa and submucosa are believed to lead to relative obstruction and work hypertrophy of the circular muscle of the pylorus. This occurs over days or weeks.[42] The fact that a "secondary" form of HPS can develop in somewhat older infants after prolonged transpyloric feeding tube presence or in patients with "congenital webs, prostaglandin-induced foveolar hyperplasia, eosinophilic gastroenteritis and antral polyps"[41] gives credence to the work hypertrophy theory. The result is an elongated pyloric length and pyloric muscle wall thickening (**Fig. 10**).[5,41,42]

The typical HPS patient presents with nonbilious projectile vomiting, vomiting with a force that allows the vomitus to cross inches if not feet. However, this forceful vomiting can occur in a refluxer, particularly if overfed and if eating ravenously. Although HPS may begin in some with what appears to be merely "spitting up," the complaint of forceful ("projectile") vomiting or continuous vomiting will cause clinical and, if necessary, imaging evaluation so as to make a rapid and correct diagnosis and avoid the

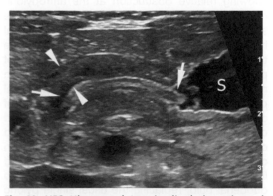

Fig. 10. HPS. Ultrasound. Longitudinal plane through pylorus. An elongated (2.2 cm) pyloric channel (marked off by *arrows*) with a thickened muscle wall (*arrowheads* mark off the muscle wall anterior to the pyloric channel) are seen, which is consistent with an ultrasonographic diagnosis of HPS. The pyloric image was unchangeable during the study, confirming the diagnosis of HPS. S, stomach.

hypochloremic metabolic alkalosis and dehydration that can occur with chronic vomiting and no treatment. Due to starvation, mild jaundice can develop in 5% of such infants.[41,42]

Severely affected infants who present with alkalosis and prolonged vomiting will look sickly and be dehydrated. The typical HPS patient, however, looks healthy, sometimes with a complaint of slower weight gain. Among experienced clinicians and surgeons, the palpation of the classic pyloric "olive," the mass of thickened and elongated pyloric muscle slightly to the right of midline, at a position just medial to the gallbladder, is pathognomonic for HPS and the classic surgery, a pyloromyotomy, can be performed.[5] Surgery will wait, in the case of the dehydrated and alkalotic patient, for rehydration and electrolyte correction. Abdominal palpation does have challenges requiring a calm infant with relaxed abdominal musculature. In addition, a distended stomach may rise anterior to the pylorus and, unless decompressed by a nasogastric tube, limit the physical examination.[47] Even with an unhindered physical examination, many physicians prefer, in these more cautious times, to seek an imaging diagnosis or at least imaging confirmation of their clinical/physical examination diagnosis.

The imaging workup for HPS is rarely aided by the plain radiograph, which is usually nonspecific. Occasionally, one may see an air-filled stomach made up several convexities, suggesting peristalsis against a relative obstruction. This image has been referred to as the caterpillar sign (see **Fig. 2**).

The two key studies that can be used to diagnose HPS are the upper GI series and pyloric ultrasound. The upper GI series diagnosis is made by showing relative obstruction at the antropyloric region noted by delay of barium flow beyond the stomach and elongated pyloric channel. Several historic signs of a positive examination include the "shoulder" sign noted by mass impression of pyloric muscle on the antrum, the "teat" sign noted by limited contrast filling of only the proximal pylorus, or the "string" sign noted by a thin line of contrast filling the abnormally long and compressed pyloric canal. Haran and colleagues[48] described the "double-track" sign of HPS. They noted two separated contrast-filled linear densities extending from antrum to duodenal bulb, replacing the usual single pyloric channel, caused by mass impression on the single pyloric channel, and resulting in two or more linear tracks of pyloric contrast material. The sign was believed specific for HPS. A *normal* upper GI shows the prepyloric antrum to be widely patent with rapid egress of barium through a pylorus no longer than a few millimeters.[5,48]

Although the upper GI series is considered an acceptable imaging modality for the diagnosis of HPS, it has shortcomings. Examinations are affected by the need to be wary of radiation exposure and fluoroscopy times. The published sensitivity of the upper GI series for the diagnosis of HPS approaches 95%, but error rates as high as 11% have been reported.[49] In addition, as with all procedural examinations, the experience and skill of the examiner are important in determining the accuracy of the results. Believe it or not, the upper GI series is as operator dependent as the diagnostic ultrasound examination.

The modern era of HPS diagnosis and antropyloric region triage analysis by ultrasound began with Teele and Smith's[50] *New England Journal of Medicine* article showing the ultrasound imaging of a pyloric olive in the transverse plane as a "doughnut" or "bagel" with an echogenic center representing mucosa and mucus surrounded by circumferential, thickened echopenic pyloric muscle (**Fig. 11**). In 1981, when Harris L. Cohen, one of the authors of this article, returned to New York from Children's Hospital National Medical Center, he had to prove to pediatric surgeons the reliability of this ultrasound diagnosis with many asking for upper GI confirmation. This was despite the recent ready availability of real-time imaging, which enhanced the ability to watch the

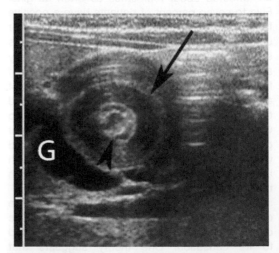

Fig. 11. Doughnut or bagel sign of HPS. Ultrasound. Axial plane through pylorus. The thick-walled pylorus (*arrow*) appears like a rounded mass in cross section. Prominent echogenic mucosa is seen centrally (*arrowhead*). The mass is what is felt on physical examination and described as a pyloric olive. The gallbladder (G) can be seen in its relatively usual anatomic relationship to the abnormal pylorus. If there were no abnormal pylorus, the gallbladder would be seen adjacent to the duodenal bulb.

antropyloric region handle swallowed or nasogastric tube–placed fluid. By 1983, the ultrasound examination had become a mainstay in the analysis of HPS, enabling rapid and direct imaging of the thickened pyloric muscle and elongated pyloric channel. Ultrasound examinations could be performed on sicker children at the bedside and without radiation exposure.

Ultrasound examination technique The ultrasound examination for neonates with possible HPS relies on a high-frequency transducer. The authors begin with a 7.5-MHz convex array probe, analyzing the layout of the SMA and SMV in relationship to the aorta and inferior vena cava to rule out an anomalous orientation associated with malrotation. If the pylorus can be clearly seen and measured without added fluid or with only the residual fluid from a prior feed, and if the findings are unchangeable, the authors may make the diagnosis without adding fluid to the stomach. The authors will, at times, allow an infant to swallow by bottle when the baby's stomach is empty and the baby is cooperative. This reveals the position of the proximal pylorus as outlined by echoless fluid. The authors often keep the patient in a right side down decubitus position during the feeding to permit rapid egress of echoless water from the patient's stomach to the duodenal bulb and descending duodenum. If food or milk products are in the stomach, the authors will remove as much as possible by an 8F-catheter 15-in nasogastric tube placed into the stomach. The authors then can place a controlled amount of fluid (usually one half of a typical feed [eg, a baby that eats 4 oz or 120 mL at a feed is given 60 mL of fluid]) into the stomach. The authors can see reflux (see **Fig. 9**) up the distal esophagus; can determine if there is any gastric or duodenal obstruction, such as a web or stenosis; and can follow the fluid to the ligament of Treitz (although not as easily as with barium on fluoroscopy). If the fluid is at the level of the duodenal bulb after crossing from right to left abdomen, the authors believe malrotation is disproven (see **Fig. 4**). The authors then look at the pylorus for an elongated length (which authors consider to be 18 mm) and a thickened muscle, which is definitively positive at 4 mm but is known to be possibly positive at greater than 3 mm. At times, the authors use a linear high-frequency transducer for better imaging of the muscle. This, however, is not necessary. If the stomach is overdistended, the pylorus can be displaced posteriorly, and the authors may use a lower frequency transducer to penetrate and image the posteriorly positioned pylorus.[42]

Classically, the ultrasound diagnosis of HPS is made using measurement and imaging criteria. Most of the measurement criteria reported in early articles on the ultrasound diagnosis of HPS have held up well to the test of time. Blumhagen and Noble[51] thought 4 mm or greater thickness of the pyloric muscle was crucial to the diagnosis of HPS. In 1986, Stunden and colleagues[52] noted that pyloric length was the most reliable measurement in diagnosing HPS from healthy patients. All their patients with HPS had a pyloric length greater than 17 mm, whereas the canal lengths for their normal patients were never more than 14 mm. The authors use an 18-mm or greater measurement as a definitively abnormal pyloric length.[42] Examiners should be wary of undermeasurement due to the curved nature of the pylorus. Straight-line measurements may undermeasure a curved structure and the authors use either a trace method to obtain the true measurement or add individual straight lines by breaking down the curve to its component straight lines and adding those up to determine true length (**Fig. 12**). Many authorities accept 3- to 4-mm pyloric wall thicknesses as abnormal. Certainly, in patients who present early (ie, within the first 4 weeks of life and particularly in patients who were born prematurely and therefore present in reality at a chronologically younger age), a wall thickness as thin as 3 mm can be positive for HPS.

In addition to measurements, ancillary visual findings are used for the diagnosis. In 1987, Cohen and colleagues[53] noted the appearance of the "ultrasonic double-track sign" in cases of HPS on ultrasound examination (**Fig. 13**). This sign is analogous to the one seen in upper GI series, and is represented on ultrasound examination by two tracks or more or echoless fluid within the pyloric channel. Ultrasound equivalents of the upper GI string sign, shoulder sign (**Fig. 14**), and other signs have also been noted. Ball and colleagues[54] use the term *cervix sign* (see **Fig. 14**) to note that the elongated hypertrophied pylorus extending from the antrum to the duodenum resembles a cervix. Thickened pyloric mucosa seen within the prepyloric antrum, which the authors called the "mucosal heaping" sign (**Fig. 15**) and which is caused by retrograde "herniation" of mucosa from constant pressure against the obstruction of HPS, has been observed ultrasonographically as well as endoscopically as a mass in the antral lumen. Reported by Hernanz-Schulman, this is called the "antral nipple" sign.[55]

According to Hernanz-Schulman and colleagues,[49] the accuracy of sonography approaches 100% for the diagnosis of HPS. Normal examinations show no pyloric muscle mass or elongated pyloric length. A hallmark of a positive ultrasound

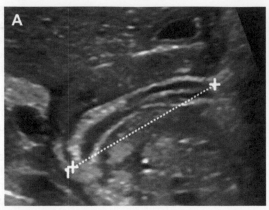
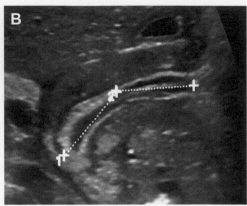

Fig. 12. Improved measuring technique for curved pyloric channel. Ultrasound. Longitudinal plane through pylorus. (*A*) Because the pyloric channel is often curved, straight measurements by ultrasound may undermeasure the true pyloric length. In this case, it was not a problem because lengths determined by all measurement methods were 2.2 cm or greater. However, an undermeasurement can sometimes result in a false-negative diagnosis. The straight measurement of a curved structure, as in this image (*dotted line*), would fall short of the true length just as a measurement of a triangle's hypotenuse would be shorter than the sum of the two other sides. (*B*) Two straight-line measurements (*two dotted lines*) obtained as components of the curve resulted in an overall length 2.5 mm greater than the 2.24 cm obtained by the single straight-line measurement (*dotted line* in *A*). At times, especially when the imager is blinded from part of the curve by, for example, an overdistended stomach partially filled with air, the differences may be even greater. 1, 1 measurement; 182, 2 measurements.

examination for HPS is the constancy of the abnormal measurements throughout the examination. If measurements are unchangeable during the examination, the diagnosis is HPS.

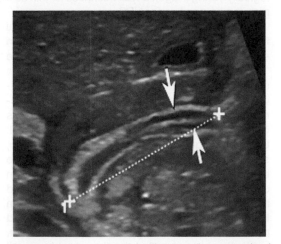

Fig. 13. Double track sign. Ultrasound. Longitudinal plane through pyloric channel. The patient has an elongated and thickened pylorus. In this case, the single channel appears to be replaced proximally by two echoless channels (*arrows*). This is simulated by mass impression on the single smooth channel, creating the appearance of two tracks. This is similar to the finding described by Haran for the upper GI series. One may see more than two channels, depending on the beam's angle through the impinged-upon channel. Dotted line indicates straight-line measurement of pylorus. Plus signs indicate each end of the pylorus. 1, 1 measurement.

Measurements that change from abnormal to normal during the ultrasound study suggest a diagnosis of pylorospasm.

Pylorospasm

Like HPS, pylorospasm is very common in infancy and a major cause of vomiting and projectile emesis. Despite this, little has been written about its ultrasound (or other) imaging. Its cause is not definitively understood. According to some theories, pylorospasm and HPS are caused by the same problems (ie, gastric hyperacidity and vagal overstimulation). Other theories suggest that pylorospasm stems from a defect in nitrous oxide production required for pyloric relaxation.[5,56]

Pylorospasm limits coordinated gastric emptying, at least transiently. In normal gastric emptying, a contraction of the gastric antrum is followed by a sequential contraction of the pyloric region and the duodenum. Contractions that inhibit a premature movement of food—while still in a more solid form—from the antrum to the duodenum are important safety mechanisms for normal physiologic actions. Pylorospasm could represent a hyperactive form of this normal physiologic action, which young infants usually outgrow.[56]

Swischuk and colleagues,[57] in discussing pylorospasm as extremely common, did not note abnormal thickening of pyloric muscle, but did indicate the need to avoid tangential imaging of the pyloric canal to avoid creating images that

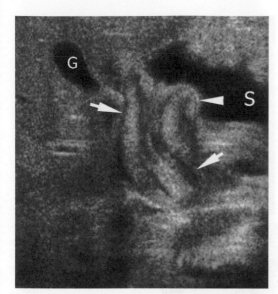

Fig. 14. Shoulder and cervix signs of HPS. Ultrasound. Longitudinal oblique plane through the pylorus. Arrowhead points to the prominent proximal pyloric muscle, which creates mass impression on the fluid-filled stomach (S) equivalent to the shoulder sign for HPS of the upper GI series. Two arrows point to the prominent shape of the abnormally thick pylorus, which looks equivalent to a cervix, and hence the designation cervix sign. G, gallbladder.

incorrectly indicate abnormal muscle-wall thickening. The authors avoid this by keeping the canal in the center of any transverse or longitudinal image used for muscle-wall measurements.

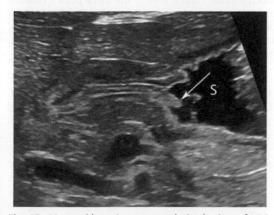

Fig. 15. Mucosal heaping or antral nipple sign of HPS. Ultrasound. Longitudinal plane through pylorus. The pylorus is thickened and elongated. Its mucosa is prominent. Just proximal to the pyloric channel, within the essentially fluid-filled stomach (S), a small soft tissue mass (*arrow*), representing herniated prominent pyloric mucosa, is seen as a mass. The authors have called this *mucosal heaping*. Hernanz-Schulman reported this as the antral nipple sign. Her paper includes an endoscopic view of this mass of mucosa.

One ultrasound study[49] of infants with suspected HPS labeled 7 of 152 as "pylorospasm or early evolving pyloric stenosis." The group had a mean pyloric muscle thickness of 2.0 mm and a mean pyloric length of 12.3 mm (range, 10–14 mm) compared with a proven HPS group with mean pyloric muscle thickness of 4.6 mm (range, 3.3–7.0 mm) and mean pyloric length of 19 mm (range, 13–29 mm). These measurements, therefore, did not overlap with those of HPS. However, others had differing experiences. Hayden and colleagues[26] had 2 of 7 gastric ulcer patients diagnosed by ultrasound with "slight thickening of the pyloric muscle" (2–3 mm), which they considered reactive hypertrophy, while 5 patients had an elongated pyloric length (1.5–2.3 cm), typical for HPS. Blumhagen[58] described cases of borderline pyloric muscle wall thickness (3–3.5 mm) that were not HPS but pylorospasm based on ultrasound evidence of occasional brief openings of the pyloric channel with peristaltic waves.

In 1998,[59] the authors reported the findings of 37 cases of HPS and 34 cases of pylorospasm proved by surgery, in the case of HPS, and by long-term clinical follow-up, in the cases of pylorospasm. Many of the pylorospasm cases had measurements overlapping those of HPS but with one difference: The abnormally long pyloric lengths and thickened pyloric muscle wall were noted for only a portion of the ultrasound examination (**Fig. 16**) with other measurements obtained during the same study *not* as long or as thick as those of HPS. Maximal wall thickness among the 34 patients with pylorospasm ranged from 1.5 to 6 mm with at least 18 patients having pyloric muscle thicknesses of 4 mm or greater—the measurement suggestive of HPS for a portion of the ultrasound study. The longest pyloric measurements obtained in that study among the 34 pylorospasm patients ranged from 3 to 27 mm, with at least 6 patients having lengths of 18 mm or more. Not only did measurements overlap but so too did visual signs. We imaged the double-track sign in many cases of pylorospasm as well as HPS. This sign is, therefore, not specific for HPS and can be visible for at least part of an ultrasound study in perhaps as many as 50% of patients with pylorospasm.[60]

Correct diagnosis of pylorospasm versus HPS is important because the respective treatments differ. Although both may present with projectile vomiting, HPS is treated with surgical pyloromyotomy while pylorospasm is treated conservatively with watchful waiting (particularly in the young infant to see if what was seen was a harbinger of HPS) and occasional use of antispasmodics.

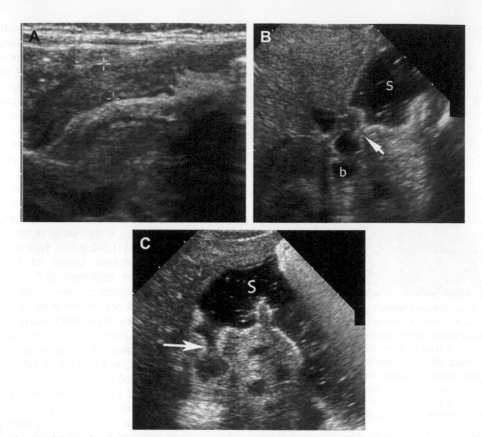

Fig. 16. Changeability of pyloric image in pylorospasm. Ultrasound. Longitudinal plane through antropyloric area. (*A*) An elongated thick-walled pylorus appears consistent with the image of a case of HPS. Graticules mark off the anterior wall's thickness. Lack of contained stomach fluid limits exact measurement of pyloric length, but approximate measurement was consistent with a positive study. (*B*) After fluid was placed into the stomach by nasogastric tube, the pylorus (*arrow*) appears much shorter. Fluid is seen in the distal pyloric channel just proximal to the fluid-filled duodenal bulb (b). (*C*) Seconds later, the pylorus opens up completely. No thick muscle is seen around the pyloric channel (*arrow*) and fluid is seen in the triangular duodenal bulb just distal to it. Such changeability from abnormal to normal or relatively normal is typical of cases of pylorospasm, which, at least for a portion of the ultrasound study, may simulate HPS. S, stomach.

With a confident diagnosis of HPS, surgery can be avoided.

To help the differentiation, the authors have over the last decade prolonged ultrasound examinations 5 to 10 minutes to help denote measurement changeability from abnormal to normal to be able to diagnose pylorospasm. Graif and colleagues[61] noted as early as 1984 that prolonging ultrasound observation for gastric content passage was a useful method for avoiding surgery in cases simulating HPS.

SUMMARY

In conclusion, clinicians must take many considerations into account when finding the causes of the various forms of neonatal vomiting. Ultrasound has been a great help in making many of these diagnoses, while also reducing radiation

exposures and occasionally obviating surgery. Clinicians who learn the techniques for ultrasound analysis of causes of vomiting will be amply rewarded and their patients will benefit.

REFERENCES

1. Cohen HL, Gilet A, Dunkin J, et al. The future of diagnostic sonography in radiology: a great imaging tool but in whose hands? In: Angtuaco T, Hamper U, Ralls P, et al, editors. Ultrasound. Practical sonography for the radiologist. Leesburg (VA): ARRS; 2009. p. 287–93.
2. Cohen HL, Babcock D, Kushner D, et al. Vomiting in infants up to 3 months of age. (ACR appropriateness criteria). Radiology 2000;215S:779–86.
3. Brenner DJ, Hall E. Computed tomography—an increasing source of radiation exposure. N Engl J Med 2007;357:2277–84.

4. Goske M, Applegate K, Boylan J, et al. The Image Gently campaign: working together to change practice. AJR Am J Roentgenol 2008;190:273–4.

5. Blumer S, Zucconi W, Cohen HL, et al. The vomiting neonate: a review of the ACR appropriateness criteria and ultrasound's role in the workup of such patients. Ultrasound Q 2004;20:79–89.

6. Durie P. Introduction to gastrointestinal imaging in pediatrics. In: Stringer D, editor. Pediatric gastrointestinal imaging. Philadelphia: BC Decker; 1989. p. 2–3.

7. Couture A. Bowel obstruction in neonates and children. In: Couture A, Baud C, Ferran J, et al, editors. Gastrointestinal tract sonography in fetuses and children. Berlin: Springer-Verlag; 2008. p. 199–204.

8. Goske M, Goldblum J, Applegate K, et al. The 'circle sign': a new sonographic sign of pneumatosis intestinalis: clinical, pathologic and experimental findings. Pediatr Radiol 1999;29:530–5.

9. Kim WY, Kim WS, Kim I, et al. Sonographic evaluation of neonates with early-stage necrotizing enterocolitis. Pediatr Radiol 2005;35:1056–61.

10. Hilton S. The child with vomiting. In: Hilton S, Edwards D, editors. Practical pediatric radiology. Philadelphia: WB Saunders; 1994. p. 297–9.

11. Alford BA, McIlhenny J. The child with acute abdominal pain and vomiting. Radiol Clin North Am 1992; 30:441–53.

12. Leonidas J, Berdon W. The gastrointestinal tract. In: Silverman F, Kuhn J, editors. Essentials of Caffey's pediatric X-ray diagnosis. Chicago: Year Book Medical Publishers; 1990. p. 1021.

13. Cohen HL. Hypertrophic pyloric stenosis. In: Cohen HL, Sivit CJ, editors. Fetal & pediatric ultrasound. A casebook approach. New York: McGraw Hill; 2001. p. 415–21.

14. Lilien LD, Srinivasan G, Pyati SP, et al. Green vomiting in the first 72 hours in normal infants. Am J Dis Child 1986;140:662–4.

15. Bowen A. The vomiting infant: recent advances and unsettled issues in imaging. Radiol Clin North Am 1988;26:377–92.

16. Hayden CK, Boulden TF, Swischuk LE, et al. Sonographic demonstration of duodenal obstruction with midgut volvulus. AJR Am J Roentgenol 1984; 143:9–10.

17. Cohen HL, Haller JO, Mestel AL, et al. Neonatal duodenum: fluid-aided US examination. Radiology 1987;164:805–9.

18. Maconi G, Radice E, Bareggi E, et al. Hydrosonography of the gastrointestinal tract. AJR Am J Roentgenol 2009;193:700–8.

19. Kraus SJ. Gastroesophageal reflux. In: Donnelly LF, editor. Diagnostic imaging: pediatrics. Salt Lake City (UT): Amirsys; 2005. p. 448–51.

20. Byrne W, D'Harlingue A. General considerations. In: Taeusch H, Ballard R, Avery M, editors. Schaffer & Avery's diseases of the newborn. 6th edition. Philadelphia: WB Saunders; 1991. p. 653–8.

21. Sivit CJ. Midgut malrotation. In: Cohen HL, Sivit CJ, editors. Fetal and pediatric ultrasound: a casebook approach. New York: McGraw Hill; 2001. p. 430–2.

22. Long FR, Kramer SS, Markowitz RI, et al. Radiographic patterns of intestinal malrotation in children. Radiographics 1996;16:547–56.

23. Weinberger E, Winters WD, Liddel RM, et al. Sonographic diagnosis of intestinal malrotation in infants: importance of the relative positions of the superior mesenteric vein and artery. AJR Am J Roentgenol 1992;159:825–8.

24. Manning PB, Murphy JP, Raynor SC, et al. Congenital diaphragmatic hernia presenting due to gastrointestinal complications. J Pediatr Surg 1992;27:1225–8.

25. Hayden CK. Gastrointestinal tract. In: Babcock DS, editor. Neonatal and pediatric ultrasonography. New York: Churchill Livingstone; 1989. p. 77–101.

26. Hayden CK, Swischuk LE, Rytting JE. Gastric ulcer disease in infants: US findings. Radiology 1987; 164:131–4.

27. O'Keefe FN, Stansberry SD, Swischuk LE, et al. Antropyloric muscle thickness at US in infants: US findings. Radiology 1991;178:827–30.

28. Ferran JL. Ultrasonographic imaging of the esophago-gastric junction. In: Couture A, Baud C, Ferran J, et al, editors. Gastrointestinal tract sonography in fetuses and children. Berlin: Springer-Verlag; 2008. p. 85–98.

29. Swischuk LE, Hayden CK, van Caillie BD. Megaaeroesophagus in children: a sign of gastroesophageal reflux. Radiology 1981;14:173–6.

30. Seibert JJ, Byrne WJ, Euler AR, et al. Gastroesophageal reflux—the acid test: scintigraphy or the pH probe? AJR Am J Roentgenol 1983;140:1087–90.

31. Heyman S, Eicher P, Alavi A. Radionuclide studies of the upper gastrointestinal tract in children with feeding disorders. J Nucl Med 1995;36:351–4.

32. Naik DR, Moore DJ. Ultrasound diagnosis of gastroesophageal reflux. Arch Dis Child 1984;59:366–7.

33. Gomes H, Lallemand A, Lallemand P. Ultrasound of the gastroesophageal junction. Pediatr Radiol 1993; 23:94–9.

34. Riccabona M, Maurer U, Lackner H, et al. The role of sonography in the evaluation of gastroesophageal reflux—correlation with pHmetry. Eur J Pediatr 1992;151:655–7.

35. McCauley RG, Darling DB, Leonidas JC, et al. Gastroesophageal reflux in infants and children: a useful classification and reliable physiologic technique for its demonstration. AJR Am J Roentgenol 1978;130:47–50.

36. Hirsch W, Kedar R, Preiss U. Color Doppler in the diagnosis of the gastroesophageal reflux children: comparison with pH measurement and B-mode ultrasound. Pediatr Radiol 1996;26:232–5.

37. Jang HS, Lee JS, Lim G, et al. Correlation of color Doppler sonographic findings with pH measurements in gastroesophageal reflux in children. J Clin Ultrasound 2001;29:212–7.

38. Veyrac C. Antro-pyloric abnormalities. In: Couture A, Baud C, Ferran J, et al, editors. Gastrointestinal tract sonography in fetuses and children. Berlin: Springer-Verlag; 2008. p. 99–129.

39. Honna T, Kamii Y, Tsuchida Y. Idiopathic gastric volvulus in infancy and childhood. J Pediatr Surg 1990;25:707–10.

40. DeGiacomo C, Maggiore G, Fiori P, et al. Chronic gastric torsion in infancy: a revisited diagnosis. Australas Radiol 1989;33:252–4.

41. Goske M, Schlesinger A. Hypertrophic pyloric stenosis. In: Slovis T, editor. Caffey's pediatric diagnostic imaging. 11th edition. Philadelphia: Mosby Elsevier; 2008. p. 2070–81.

42. Haller JO, Cohen HL. Hypertrophic pyloric stenosis: diagnosis using US. Radiology 1986;161:335–9.

43. Schechter R, Torfs CP, Bateson TF. The epidemiology of infantile hypertrophic pyloric stenosis. Pediatr Perinatal Epidemiol 1997;11:407–27.

44. Oue T, Puri P. Smooth muscle cell hypertrophy versus hyperplasia in infantile hypertrophic pyloric stenosis. Pediatr Res 1999;45:853–7.

45. Spitz L, Zail SS. Serum gastrin levels in congenital hypertrophic pyloric stenosis. J Pediatr Surg 1976;11:33–5.

46. Dodge JA, Karim AA. Induction of pyloric hypertrophy by pentagastrin: an animal model for infantile hypertrophic pyloric stenosis. Gut 1976;17:280–4.

47. Hernanz–Schulman M. Infantile hypertrophic pyloric stenosis. Radiology 2003;227:319–31.

48. Haran PJ, Darling DB, Sciammas F. The value of the double-track sign as a differentiating factor between pylorospasm and hypertrophic pyloric stenosis in infants. Radiology 1966;86:723–5.

49. Hernanz–Schulman M, Sells LL, Ambrosino MM, et al. Hypertrophic pyloric stenosis in the infant without a palpable olive: accuracy of sonographic diagnosis. Radiology 1994;193:771–6.

50. Teele RL, Smith EH. Ultrasound in the diagnosis of idiopathic hypertrophic pyloric stenosis. N Engl J Med 1977;296:1149–50.

51. Blumhagen JD, Noble HGS. Muscle thickness in hypertrophic pyloric stenosis: sonographic determination. AJR Am J Roentgenol 1983;140:221–3.

52. Stunden RJ, LeQuesne GW, Little KET. The improved ultrasound diagnosis of hypertrophic pyloric stenosis. Pediatr Radiol 1986;16:200–5.

53. Cohen HL, Schechter S, Mestel A, et al. Ultrasonic "double track" sign in hypertrophic pyloric stenosis. J Ultrasound Med 1987;6:139–43.

54. Ball TI, Atkinson GO Jr, Gay BB. Ultrasound diagnosis of hypertrophic pyloric stenosis: real-time application and the demonstration of a new sonographic sign. Radiology 1983;147:499–502.

55. Hernanz–Schulman M, Dinauer P, Ambrosino MM, et al. The antral nipple sign of pyloric mucosal prolapse: endoscopic correlation of a new sonographic observation in patients with pyloric stenosis. J Ultrasound Med 1995;14:283–7.

56. Cohen HL. Pylorospasm. In: Dachman A, Ralls P, Cohen HL, editors. Gastrointestinal disease (Sixth Series) test and syllabus. Baltimore (MD): American College of Radiology Publications- Cenveo; 2004. p. 1–11.

57. Swischuk L, Hayden CK Jr, Stansberry S. Sonographic pitfalls in imaging of the antropyloric region in infants. Radiographics 1989;9:437–47.

58. Blumhagen J. Invited commentary: the role of ultrasonography in the evaluation of vomiting in infants. Pediatr Radiol 1986;16:267.

59. Cohen HL, Zinn H, Haller J, et al. Ultrasonography of pylorospasm: findings may simulate hypertrophic pyloric stenosis. J Ultrasound Med 1998;17:705–12.

60. Cohen HL, Blumer SL, Zucconi WB. The ultrasonic double-track sign: not pathognomonic for hypertrophic pyloric stenosis—can be seen in pylorospasm. J Ultrasound Med 2004;23:641–6.

61. Graif M, Itzchak Y, Avigad I, et al. The pylorus in infancy: overall sonographic assessment. Pediatr Radiol 1984;14:14–7.

Ultrasound of the Acute Abdomen in Children

Marthe M. Munden, MD[a,b,*], Jeanne G. Hill, MD[c]

KEYWORDS

- Pancreatitis • Appendicitis • Infectious colitis
- Duplication cysts • Intussusception

In the setting of the acute abdomen in the pediatric population, ultrasound has proven to be an extremely effective and readily available diagnostic tool, requiring no patient preparation or radiation exposure. The advent of newer and higher-resolution probes has added to the diagnostic capability. Individual experience in an imaging center or hospital determines the level of comfort in using ultrasound to determine the etiology of acute abdominal symptoms—from the simple diagnosis of hypertrophic pyloric stenosis to diagnosis and treatment of ileocolic intussusception using ultrasound guidance. This article reviews techniques and findings during sonographic investigation in the emergency department setting of acute abdominal pain.

MIDGUT VOLVULUS IN THE OLDER CHILD

Midgut volvulus secondary to malrotation typically presents in the neonatal period with bilious emesis, and diagnosis often is made by an upper gastrointestinal contrast examination (UGI). However, patients beyond the neonatal period with vague symptoms such as malabsorption and chronic diarrhea related to unsuspected nonobstructive midgut volvulus may present for ultrasound examination.[1] In those patients, a curvilinear or linear probe can be used to evaluate the epigastric region, revealing a distended stomach and duodenum ending in a beak-like configuration with an associated whirlpool sign, which represents the jejunal vein circling clockwise around the superior mesenteric artery (SMA) (**Fig. 1**). The superior mesenteric vein (SMV) may be found to lie anterior or to the left of the SMA with malrotation, although a normal SMA/SMV relationship does not exclude malrotation. Additionally, vessel inversion can be seen with normal gut rotation (**Fig. 2**). Recent publications have reported that the third portion of the duodenum is always found to be intraperitoneal at surgery for malrotation/midgut volvulus, and finding the third portion of the duodenum positioned in the retroperitoneal space between the SMA and aorta in the sagittal and transverse planes sonographically excludes malrotation.[2,3] Although many still feel more comfortable excluding malrotation with a UGI, the sonographic documentation of a normal retroperitoneal position of the transverse duodenum is becoming routine in some centers.

PANCREATITIS

Abdominal pain caused by acute pancreatitis is not uncommon in major pediatric emergency centers. Patients with acute pancreatitis usually present with nausea and vomiting, acute onset of epigastric pain that may radiate to the back, and epigastric tenderness. Serum amylase levels can

a Pediatric Radiology Department, Children's Health System of Alabama, Alabama Children's Hospital, 1600 7th Avenue South, Birmingham, AL 35233, USA
b Edward B. Singleton Department of Diagnostic Imaging, Texas Children's Hospital, 6621 Fannin Street, MC2-2521, Houston, TX 77030, USA
c Department of Radiology and Radiological Science, Medical University of South Carolina, 96 Jonathan Lucas Street, Suite 210, Clinical Science Building, MSC 323, Charleston, SC 29425, USA
* Corresponding author. Pediatric Radiology Department, Children's Health System of Alabama, Alabama Children's Hospital, 1600 7th Avenue South, Birmingham, AL 35233.
E-mail address: mmmunden@texaschildrens.org

Ultrasound Clin 5 (2010) 113–135
doi:10.1016/j.cult.2009.11.016
1556-858X/10/$ – see front matter © 2010 Elsevier Inc. All rights reserved.

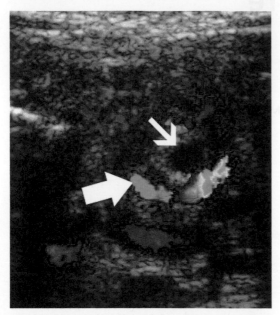

Fig. 1. Malrotation with midgut volvulus. Transverse image shows the jejunal vein (*thicker arrow*) circling the SMA (*slender arrow*), representing the whirlpool sign. Incomplete obstruction caused by midgut volvulus was found at surgery.

be normal with severe pancreatitis, and hyperamylasemia is not specific for pancreatic disease.[4] Diagnosis requires at least a threefold elevation of serum pancreatic enzymes. Etiologies for acute

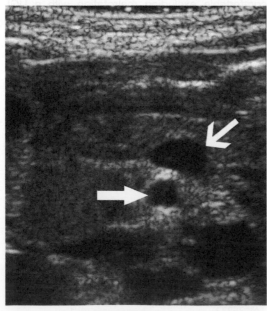

Fig. 2. Abnormal SMA/SMV position. Transverse sonographic image shows the SMV (*slender arrow*) located anterior to the SMA (*thicker arrow*).

pancreatitis in pediatrics include trauma, gallstones, systemic infections, anatomic abnormalities of the pancreaticobiliary system, medications including immunosuppressive drug therapy, hereditary pancreatitis, and congenital anomalies at the pancreaticobiliary junction including duodenal duplication cysts. A recurrence rate of 9% for pancreatitis is reported in children.[5]

The normal pancreas in children is often clearly visible sonographically in the fasting patient and is homogeneously isoechoic to slightly hyperechoic to the liver in slender patients (**Fig. 3**). In patients with a larger body habitus, the pancreas is hyperechoic to the liver, as obesity is associated with increasing fatty accumulation within the pancreas.[6] The left lobe of the liver serves as an acoustic window. If necessary, and if the patient is able, the stomach can be filled with water to provide an acoustic window.

Ultrasound findings in acute pancreatitis include focal or diffuse pancreatic enlargement with decreased distinction of pancreatic margins, heterogeneous echotexture, and peripancreatic fluid collections. The pancreas can be normal in appearance in mild pancreatitis.[7] Chao and colleagues found a significant association between acute pancreatitis and a dilated pancreatic duct (>1.5 mm from ages 1 to 6 years, >1.9 mm from ages 7 to 12, or >2.2 mm in the older child) (**Fig. 4**).[8] In the setting of acute epigastric pain with either sonographic or clinical findings suggesting pancreatitis, the right upper quadrant should be evaluated for presence or absence of gallstones, choledocholithiasis, choledochal cysts, and even duplication cysts which could lead to pancreatitis (**Fig. 5**).[9,10] Ultrasound is useful to assess complications of pancreatitis such as

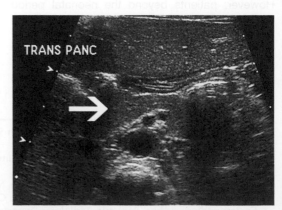

TRANS PANC

Fig. 3. Normal pancreas. Transverse sonographic image showing a normal pancreas (*arrow*), isoechoic to the liver, in a 10-year-old child. Note distinct margins and homogenous echogenicity.

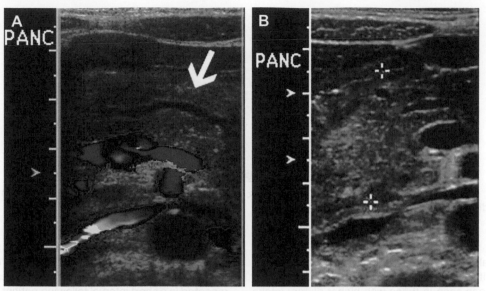

Fig. 4. Acute pancreatitis in a 10-year-old male. (*A*) Transverse image using linear transducer shows a mildly dilated pancreatic duct (*arrow*). (*B*) Transverse image shows enlargement and heterogeneously increased echogenicity of the pancreatic head (between cursors).

pseudocyst formation, pseudoaneurysms, and splenic vein thrombosis (**Fig. 6**). In the setting of traumatic pancreatic injury, computed tomography (CT) is preferred in the acute setting. Follow-up often can be performed sonographically to watch for development for peripancreatic fluid collections and traumatic pancreatitis. Endoscopic ultrasound is also emerging as a valuable tool to evaluate pancreatic biliary disease in children.[11,12] Magnetic resonance (MR) cholangiopancreatography is not performed by most centers in the setting of an acute abdomen.

APPENDICITIS

Appendicitis remains one of the most common indications for surgery in the pediatric population, and complications caused by delayed patient presentation remain prevalent. Appendicitis occurs more commonly in developed countries and has a peak incidence in males from 10 to 14 years of age, and females from 15 to 19 years of age, the time at which lymphoid follicles lining the appendix reach their maximum size.[13] Proposed etiologies for lumen obstruction of the appendix include lymphoid hyperplasia (possibly

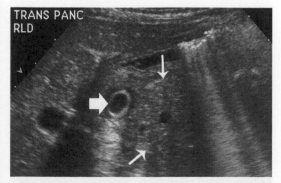

Fig. 5. Duodenal duplication cyst causing pancreatitis in a 2-year-old child. Transverse image shows diffuse enlargement of the pancreatic head (*between slender arrows*) secondary to a duodenal duplication cyst (*short arrow*).

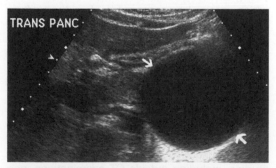

Fig. 6. Pancreatic pseudocyst complicating first episode of acute pancreatitis in a 10-year-old girl. Transverse ultrasound image showing a poorly defined pseudocyst containing internal debris (*between arrows*) adjacent to the pancreatic tail.

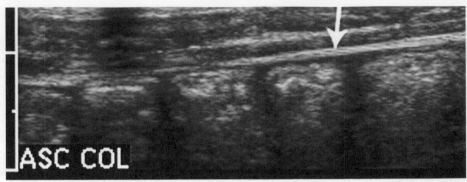

Fig. 7. Normal ascending colon. Sagittal sonographic image shows normal haustral markings (*arrow*) of the ascending colon.

of viral etiology), dehydration, fecaliths, and even parasites. A decreased incidence of appendicitis has been seen in those with higher dietary intake of fiber.[14] Symptoms can be vague, with less than half presenting with the classic scenario of insidious onset of abdominal pain migrating from the periumbilical region to the right lower quadrant (RLQ) associated with nausea and anorexia.[15] Diarrhea is not typically seen unless there is perforation and peritonitis, more often occurring in the young patient under 3 years of age, frequently confused with gastroenteritis, which may lead to a delay in diagnosis.[16]

The rate of appendiceal perforation is significantly greater in children presenting with symptoms for more than 24 hours.[17] Unfortunately, the probability of appendiceal perforation is highest in those with more limited ability to communicate. The incidence of perforation has been shown to be about 60% for a 3-year-old child, 50% for a 5-year-old child, and this incidence decreases with increasing age.[18] The omentum is also underdeveloped in the very young and unable to contain purulent material, which may be responsible for the diffuse peritonitis often present with perforated appendicitis in small children. Appendicitis is rare in neonates and infants, possibly because of the funnel shape of the appendix in infancy, which reduces the possibility of luminal obstruction.[14,19]

Ultrasound evaluation of RLQ pain is an excellent tool, as appendicitis and its mimics commonly present in the pediatric emergency department. It is not unusual to find multiple prior radiologic studies, including outside CT examinations, performed over a several year period in a single patient for abdominal pain, which can lead to high-accumulated radiation doses if CT is used repeatedly. If necessary, with an equivocal initial

ultrasound examination and continued clinical concern for appendicitis, ultrasound can be repeated in a short interval following patient observation without the risk of additional radiation.

At the beginning of the ultrasound examination, it is quite useful to ask the child to use a finger to point to the area where it hurts the most. Even the youngest of patients usually can comply. History obtained during the ultrasound examination is helpful in determining if the pain is more of a chronic nature, suggestive of possible inflammatory bowel disorder, acute with minimal emesis as in appendicitis, or associated with diarrhea in an older child, more typical of gastroenteritis. Using a high-resolution linear transducer with continued, gradual compression to displace bowel loops (the technique described by Puylaert), the area indicated by the patient should be examined first.[20] If the appendix is not found readily, slow, gradual compression is used to locate the borders of the ascending colon (**Fig. 7**), identified by position

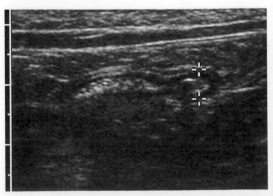

Fig. 8. Normal appendix. Transverse image of the right lower quadrant (RLQ) shows normal gut signature of a normal appendix, including the tip (*between cursors*).

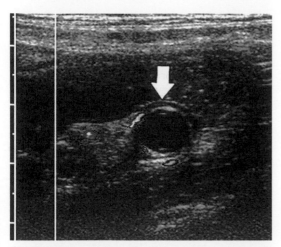

Fig. 9. Acute appendicitis. Transverse sonographic image of the RLQ shows a distended appendix with intact mucosa (*arrow*), hyperemia, but no surrounding inflammatory changes in this 9-year-old child with onset of pain less than 24 hours.

and detectable haustral folds. The transducer is moved caudally to find the cecum and terminal ileum, identified by its compressibility, peristaltic activity, and lack of a blind tip termination. The appendix arises from the cecal tip 1 to 2 cm below the origin of the terminal ileum. Additional techniques, such as using the opposite hand to compress posteriorly while scanning anteriorly, as well as placing the patient in the left lateral decubitus position to displace the cecum and appendix more medially, can be useful.[21]

The appendix is retrocecal in location in 28% to 68% of patients at surgery and autopsy and within the pelvis in 12.8% to 53% of cases.[14,22] When the appendix is retrocecal and extraperitoneal, patients may have less focal abdominal pain and more flank pain, which can lead to difficulty in diagnosis. Baldiserotto and Marchiori have shown success in finding the retrocecal appendix by examining the right flank transversely using a curvilinear transducer starting from the edge of the liver to the iliac crest, then longitudinally from the axillary line continuing posteriorly to the lumbar region. For a deep pelvic location, a curvilinear transducer can be used scanning through a distended bladder, followed by a linear transducer with graded compression after voiding if a dilated appendix is not found.[22]

The normal appendix is a slender tubular structure with preserved gut signature, easily compressible with no hyperemia, and a mean diameter of 0.39 cm (**Fig. 8**). The appendiceal lumen of the normal appendix may be empty or filled with fecal material, gas, or both. In some centers experienced in gastrointestinal (GI) ultrasound, the normal appendix has been found in up to 82% of children.[23]

In about 5% of cases, inflammation is confined to the appendiceal tip, making examination of the entire appendix and identifying the tip important.[24,25] The sonographic diagnosis of appendicitis can be made when a reproducible fluid-filled, noncompressible, distended tubular structure is found that measures greater than 6 mm in diameter with calipers placed at the outer borders of the muscularis propria (**Fig. 9**). The inflamed appendix may contain a shadowing fecalith, causing sharply defined posterior acoustic shadowing. Hyperemia of the wall of the appendix has been shown to be a sensitive indicator of inflammation, helpful in borderline cases.[26] With increasing

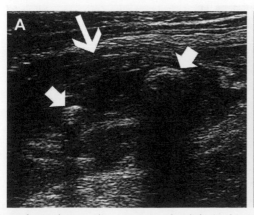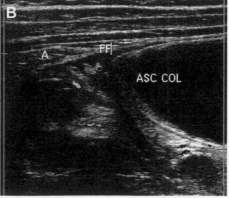

Fig. 10. Perforated appendix containing fecaliths in this 7-year-old boy with onset of pain 3 days prior. (*A*) Ultrasound image shows loss of gut signature in this distended appendix (*slender arrow*) containing two shadowing fecaliths (*short arrows*). (*B*) Transverse image shows appendix (*A*) and small amount of free fluid (FF) lateral to the dilated ascending colon.

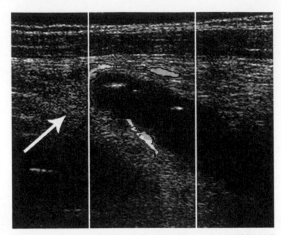

Fig. 11. Omental fat surrounding a perforated appendix. Transverse image through the RLQ shows a distended, hyperemic appendix surrounded by echogenic omental fat (*arrow*) in this patient with 3 days of pain and a perforated appendix at surgery.

inflammation from obstruction, loss of venous outflow and wall ischemia develops, causing loss of the normally visible alternating layers of the normal gut signature (**Fig. 10**). Bacterial invasion of the appendiceal wall, and thrombosis of the appendicular artery and veins, eventually lead to gangrene and perforation of the appendix. Echogenic surrounding omental fat and adjacent pericecal or periappendiceal free fluid develops, suggesting appendiceal perforation (**Fig. 11**).[27,28] In the absence of a visualized appendix because of perforation, hyperechoic mesenteric fat, RLQ and pelvic fluid collections, dilated small bowel, and a free-floating fecalith can be strong indicators of inflammation caused by a ruptured appendix (**Fig. 12**).[29,30]

Treatment for perforated appendicitis is controversial, and information regarding the location, size, and complexity of abscess collections, and presence or absence of a fecalith, provide necessary information for decisions in management. These should be evaluated sonographically at presentation.[31,32] When indicated, additional CT imaging is used.

An exception to the accepted diameter for an inflamed appendix includes patients with cystic fibrosis (CF). The incidence of appendicitis in CF is 1% to 2%, lower than the general population (7%), and the diameter of the compressed appendix identified in CF patients without appendicitis has been shown to be greater than 6 mm in both the pediatric and adult populations.[33]

Although initial evaluation for appendicitis with ultrasound is preferred in many centers, obesity and the individual experience of an imaging center may help determine which patient undergoes an ultrasound and which patient would benefit from initial evaluation with CT.

APPENDICITIS IN THE VERY YOUNG

As mentioned previously, appendicitis occurs less frequently in the young child, but the perforation rate is high.[18] Abscess formation is much more likely in children under 5 years of age than in older children. One must keep appendicitis in mind when examining a young child with symptoms of gastroenteritis lasting longer than expected. Inflammation from an underlying ruptured appendix can lead to unusual clinical presentations such as a failure to bear weight, flank pain

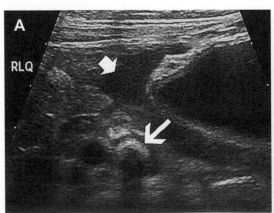
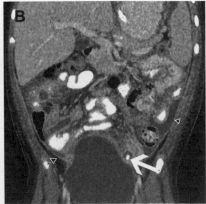

Fig. 12. Multiple abscesses complicating a perforated appendix in a 23-month-old. (*A*) A transverse image of the RLQ shows echogenic free fluid (*short arrow*) containing a free-floating fecalith (*slender arrow*). CT coronal reformatted image obtained 3 days later (*B*) showing fecalith now located left lower quadrant (LLQ) (*arrow*) and multiple abscess collections (*arrow heads*) throughout the abdomen.

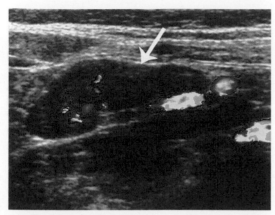

Fig. 13. Mesenteric adenitis. Transverse image of the RLQ showing prominent, mildly hyperemic lymph nodes (*arrow*) caused by mesenteric adenitis. A normal appendix was present.

with fever, and scrotal swelling in the very young.[16,18,19,34]

GI PATHOLOGY THAT MAY MIMIC APPENDICITIS

Mesenteric adenitis is one of the most common alternate diagnoses made during evaluation for suspected appendicitis.[35] Primary mesenteric adenitis has been defined as a self-limiting inflammation of RLQ mesenteric nodes with three or more lymph nodes 5 mm or greater in short axis diameter, and the presence of a normal appendix (**Fig. 13**). In secondary mesenteric adenitis, a specific inflammatory process is present such as infectious colitis, Crohn disease, or ulcerative colitis.[36] Infectious colitis may be caused *Yersinia enterocolitica*, *Campylobacter jejuni*, *Salmonella*, or other organisms.[37,38] It is important to identify

a normal appendix, as lymph nodes also can be enlarged with appendicitis.

With viral gastroenteritis, findings are nonspecific but may include a fluid-filled colon, small amounts of ascites. Findings, however, usually do not include intestinal wall thickening (>1.5 mm in the terminal ileum or >2 mm in the colon).[39] Ultrasound findings with bacterial ileocolitis caused by *Yersinia*, *Campylobacter*, *Salmonella*, and other organisms include wall thickening of the terminal ileum and cecum with hyperemia and adjacent enlarged lymph nodes (**Fig. 14**). A small amount of ascites is often present, but the surrounding fat is not inflamed.[40,41] Although these findings are nonspecific as to the underlying etiology, they can provide an alternate diagnosis and help to exclude appendicitis.

In the setting of abdominal pain with bloody diarrhea in a young child, the finding of wall thickening of the colon may represent the intestinal prodrome, which precedes the hematologic and renal manifestations of hemolytic–uremic syndrome (HUS). The involvement of the colon varies from segmental to diffuse, with the transverse colon most frequently involved. Small bowel loops can be involved along with mesenteric inflammatory changes. The clinical history is crucial for diagnosis as HUS occurs a few days after ingestion of contaminated or undercooked ground meat containing *Escherichia coli* O157:H7, *Shigella*, *Campylobacter*, and other organisms.[42–44]

INFLAMMATORY BOWEL DISEASE

Bowel wall thickening is a nonspecific sonographic finding that can be seen with infectious, inflammatory, and ischemic bowel disease. The degree of wall thickening and distribution of

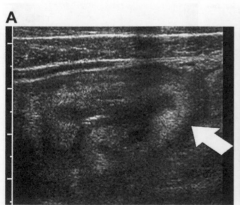
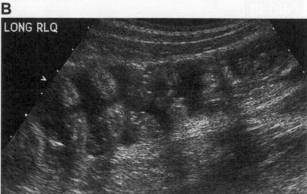

Fig. 14. Bacterial enteritis. (*A*) Ultrasound showing marked wall thickening of the cecum (*arrow*) in a child with RLQ pain, which returned to normal (*B*) 4 days later. Stool cultures were positive for enterohemorrhagic *Escherichia coli*.

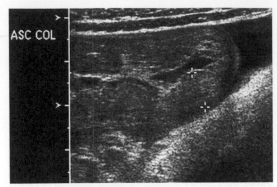

Fig. 15. Marked wall thickening of the ascending colon (*cursors*) with loss of normal layer stratification in this patient presenting with RLQ pain, later diagnosed as Crohn disease.

affected bowel vary between Crohn disease, ulcerative colitis (UC), and other nonviral GI disease. In the acute setting, ultrasound is helpful in determining the location and extent of bowel disease, which in context with clinical information, can lead to a diagnosis or differential diagnosis.[45] Although controversial, increased bowel wall thickness with loss of the normal layer stratification of hypoechoic mucosa and muscularis mucosa, echogenic submucosa, and hypoechoic muscularis propria is felt by some to correlate with the severity of inflammation with inflammatory bowel disease (IBD).[39]

Crohn disease is a transmural inflammation of the affected bowel that results in severe bowel wall thickening, inflammation of the fat surrounding the ileum and cecum, mesenteric adenopathy, and bowel loop separation. The target sign is the classic sonographic finding described in Crohn disease with transverse images of affected bowel showing a strong echogenic center and surrounding hypoechoic rim.[45] The involved areas are mainly small bowel and ascending colon, with a mural thickness ranging from 9 to 10 mm (**Fig. 15**).[46] With chronic disease, the bowel wall is thickened and typically hypoechoic because of fibrosis. Complications of Crohn disease include abscess formation, bowel obstruction, and fistula formation. Gas bubbles may be seen within fistulous tracts.[47] Up to one third of patients with Crohn disease involving the ileocecal region present with acute symptoms that mimic appendicitis.[48] The appendix itself can be involved with Crohn disease, seen in 21% of patients in a series reported by Ripolles and colleagues (**Fig. 16**).[49] All of their patients with appendiceal involvement by Crohn disease also had associated thickening of the terminal ileum or cecum, which helped differentiate the findings from acute appendicitis.

Diffuse wall thickening is also seen with ulcerative colitis, but the thickness of the ileum has been noted to be about 5 mm, while the colon wall thickness was greater. Range of mural wall thickness of the colon in UC has been shown to be a little wider, 7 mm to 10 mm, and overall less prominent than that of Crohn disease, with preserved wall stratification in UC.[45,46] Sonographic features that may help differentiate between Crohn disease and UC include location of bowel wall thickening, with presence of skip lesions and pericolic abscess more likely in Crohn disease. With underlying severe disease, ultrasound is less risky than direct visualization in searching for areas of bowel involvement.

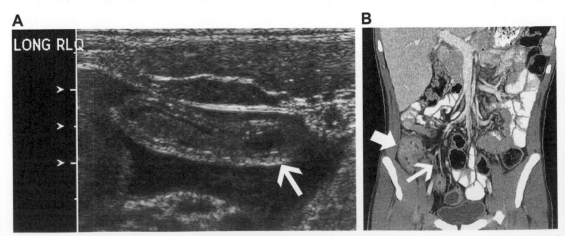

Fig. 16. Distended appendix caused by Crohn disease. (*A*) Ultrasound RLQ shows a thickened appendix (*arrow*) with surrounding ascites due to Crohn disease with coronal reformatted CT (*B*) showing enhancing appendix (*slender arrow*) with inflammation of ascending colon and cecum (*short arrow*).

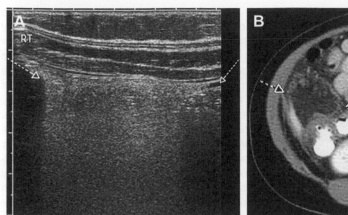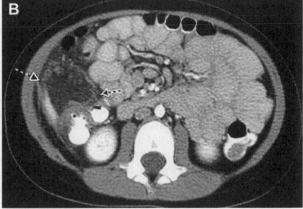

Fig. 17. Omental infarction. (*A*) Ultrasound shows diffuse echogenicity (*between arrows*) within the anterior abdomen just medial to the ascending colon, confirmed by CT (*B*) showing inflammation caused by infarcted omentum (*between arrows*).

OMENTAL INFARCTION

Omental infarction, a rare cause for acute abdominal pain, is more common in adults, but about 15% of cases present in the pediatric population. Symptoms include pain localized to the right upper or lower quadrant of a few days' duration, but associated nausea and vomiting are rare.[50] The pathogenesis is unknown, and it may occur with or without torsion of the omentum. Predisposing factors may include kinking of veins or venous congestion following a large meal, venous insufficiency caused by trauma, or thrombosis of omental veins.[51,52] Additional predisposing factors

include strenuous activity and obesity, which is increasing in the childhood population.

Ultrasound findings include an ovoid, hyperechoic soft tissue mass located between the anterior abdominal wall and transverse or ascending colon with few vessels within the mass and peripheral hyperemia (**Fig. 17**).[53] A less common appearance includes a hyperechoic mass containing an avascular hypoechoic tubular structure, which has been found to represent twisted, infarcted omental tissue at gross pathology.[51] Some advocate surgical treatment, and others recommend a conservative approach to therapy.

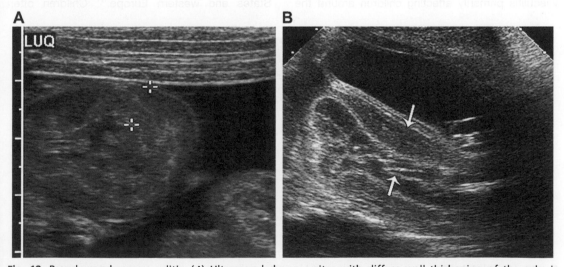

Fig. 18. Pseudomembranous colitis. (*A*) Ultrasound shows ascites with diffuse wall thickening of the splenic flexure (*between cursors*) and (*B*) rectum (*arrows*) compatible with pancolonic involvement of pseudomembranous colitis.

PSEUDOMEMBRANOUS COLITIS

Pseudomembranous colitis (PMC) is associated with a prior course of antibiotics or other agents that allow superinfection with *Clostridium difficile*. In the preantibiotic era, PMC was associated with shock, uremia, heavy metal intoxication, and cardiovascular disease. The enterotoxin of *C difficile* causes a severe inflammatory response within the colon. Symptoms of PMC typically occur after about 4 days of antibiotic therapy but have been reported to occur as long as 6 weeks later. Patients present with watery diarrhea, severe abdominal pain, fever, and leukocytosis. Diagnosis is made with detection of *C difficile* in the stool, tissue culture assay for toxin B, or antigen detection in the stool by rapid enzyme immunoassays.[54]

PMC causes the formation of yellow plaques, or pseudo membranes adherent to the gut mucosa and is generally a pancolitis, although at times involvement is more segmental.[47] Plain film findings of generalized thumb printing throughout the colon are typical, representing the striking thickening of the colon wall. Ultrasound findings include marked thickening of a hypoechoic mucosal layer with narrowing of the gut lumen and thickened echogenic submucosa representing the plaque formation with associated edema. The hypoechoic outer layer of muscularis propria is normal and thin. Ascites is present in up to 77% of those with PMC (**Fig. 18**).[55]

HENOCH-SCHONLEIN PURPURA

Henoch-Schonlein purpura (HSP) is a systemic vasculitis primarily affecting children around the age of 4, although persons of any age can be affected. Pediatric cases often are preceded by a viral or bacterial infection. The etiology is uncertain, but it represents a disorder of the immune response with immune complexes deposited in glomerular capillaries and small blood vessels of the skin, GI tract, and other organs.[56] Clinically, patients present with a petechial or purpuric rash, more commonly involving the lower extremities, arthritis, and nephritis. Abdominal pain caused by hemorrhage and edema of bowel occurs in 50% to 60% of patients. The abdominal pain may precede or follow the rash. The duodenum and small bowel are the most frequent sites of involvement of the GI tract in HSP. Bowel wall thickening caused by vasculitis-associated ischemia has a mean thickness of 9 mm and involves longer segments than bowel thickening associated with hematoma (**Fig. 19**).[57,58] Echogenic thickening of the mucosa and submucosa tends to be circumferential in the areas of ischemia. Asymmetric bowel wall thickening can be seen with associated intramural hematoma, sometimes confused with intussusception, a well-known complication of HSP.[59] Free peritoneal fluid is commonly present.

LYMPHOMA

The most frequent site of non-Hodgkin lymphoma involvement in children is the GI tract, affecting distal ileum, cecum, appendix, and ascending colon most frequently.[60] Burkitt's lymphoma is a highly aggressive type of non-Hodgkin lymphoma that commonly affects children. The nonendemic, sporadic form of Burkitt lymphoma accounts for up to 40% of lymphoma in children in the United States and western Europe.[61] Children often

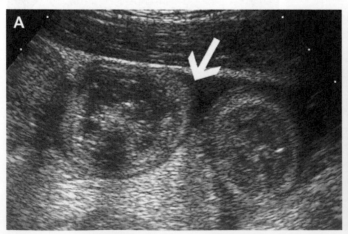
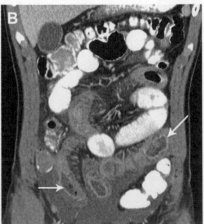

Fig. 19. Henoch-Schonlein purpura in a 16-year-old boy presenting with abdominal pain and petechial rash. (*A*) Sagittal ultrasound image shows more moderate wall thickening of small bowel with ascites. (*B*) Coronal CT shows long segments of thickened, enhancing, fluid filled small bowel (*arrows*).

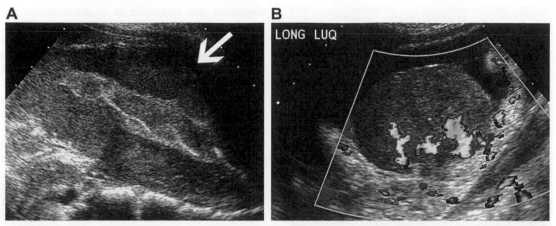

Fig. 20. Lymphoma. (*A*) Sagittal ultrasound image shows diffuse and marked bowel wall thickening (*arrow*) and (*B*) hyperemic solid mass surrounded by ascites in this 3-year-old child presenting with abdominal pain caused by lymphoma.

present with abdominal pain or lower abdominal mass, with vomiting, GI bleeding, or possible secondary intussusceptions. Symptoms may be confused with appendicitis. The tumor spreads throughout the submucosa and can be seen sonographically as severe hypoechoic bowel wall thickening with loss of normal stratification of layers (**Fig. 20**). A focal mass with large hypoechoic areas may be seen in areas with secondary tumor necrosis. The bowel lumen may be narrowed because of tumor infiltration.[62] Enlarged mesenteric nodes may be seen.

INTUSSUSCEPTION

Intussusception, an invagination or telescoping of bowel into an adjacent segment of distal bowel (**Fig. 21**), is a common pediatric abdominal emergency with a reported incidence of 56 cases per

100,000 hospitalizations per year in the United States.[63] The so-called idiopathic ileocolic intussusceptions arise from the ileum secondary to hyperplasia of the Peyer's patches and typically present with intermittent, colicky abdominal pain. The usual age at presentation is 5 months to 3 years, with peak incidence between the ages of 5 and 9 months.[64] The development of an intussusception in patients outside of this age range suggests an underlying pathologic lead point, either from a focal or diffuse abnormality of the GI tract.[65]

Clinical presentation is highly variable. The classic triad of intermittent abdominal pain,

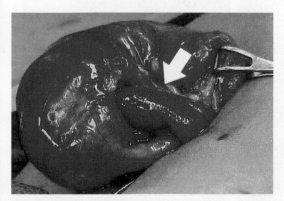

Fig. 21. Intussusception. Intraoperative image demonstrating an ileocolic intussusception with intussuscepted loop and mesenteric fat (*arrow*) entering intussuscipiens.

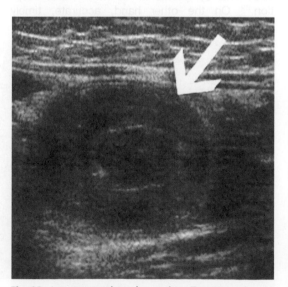

Fig. 22. Intussusception, donut sign. Transverse image of the apex of the intussusception (*arrow*) shows the hypoechoic donut.

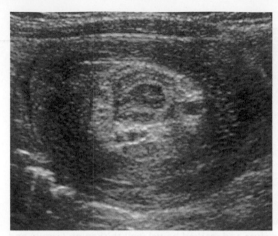

Fig. 23. Intussusception, crescent-in-donut sign. A crescent of echogenic mesenteric fat surrounds the central intussusceptum.

vomiting and right upper quadrant abdominal mass has a positive predictive value of 93%, increasing to 100% with the addition of rectal bleeding.[66] The triad of colicky abdominal pain, abdominal mass and currant jelly stools, however, occurs in less than 50% of patients, and symptoms frequently overlap with other etiologies, making clinical diagnosis difficult.[67,68] In addition to the characteristic pain, other clinical features at presentation may include irritability, bilious vomiting, bloody stools, and lethargy. Should lethargy predominate, initial misdiagnosis of a central nervous system abnormality is not uncommon. In fact, as many as 70% of the children with these abdominal symptoms fail to have intussusception.[69] On the other hand, accurate, timely

diagnosis and treatment of intussusception are important, as delay may result in obstruction, bowel ischemia, perforation and peritonitis, and rarely, death.[67] Therefore, clinicians rely on imaging to confirm or exclude the presence of intussusception.

In many institutions, ultrasound has emerged as the initial imaging modality of choice, replacing the diagnostic contrast enema, in patients with clinically suspected intussusception.[67,70–72] Several studies have verified the reliability of ultrasound as a screening examination for intussusception, with published sensitivity of 97% to 100% and specificity of 88% to 100%, even in the hands of appropriately trained residents and fellows.[73–77] Additionally, in the absence of intussusception, sonography may identify or exclude alternative pathology.[66,68]

Sonograms for intussusception should be performed with a high-frequency (5 to 10 MHz) linear transducer focusing on colon and small bowel. Ileocolic intussusceptions are not subtle masses, measuring several centimeters in diameter. Typically, the intussusceptions are localized just deep to the abdominal wall on the right in the subhepatic region, but they may be found in all quadrants of the abdomen, from cecum to rectum.

Several signs have been coined to describe the variable sonographic patterns of intussusception including the doughnut, target, bulls eye, and multiple concentric ring signs on transverse imaging and pseudokidney, sandwich, and hayfork signs on longitudinal imaging.[72,78–81] In fact, pathologic correlation has revealed that the sonographic appearance depends on the length of the intussusception, the part of the intussusception

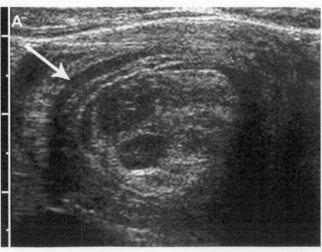
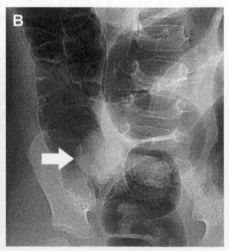

Fig. 24. Intussusception reduction. (*A*) Transverse ultrasound image shows easily identified concentric rings of bowel wall in this easily reduced intussusception. (*B*) Intussusception being reduced through ileocecal valve (*arrow*).

being scanned, and the degree of ischemia in the intussusception.[76]

On axial scanning of the leading edge or apex of the intussusception, the intussuscipiens and everted limb of the intussusceptum create a peripheral hypoechoic ring separated from the hypoechoic central limb of the intussusceptum by serosa, producing the doughnut sign (**Fig. 22**). More proximally, the intussusception has multiple concentric layers. From outside in, the layers consist of: 1) the thin hypoechoic outer bowel wall of the intussuscipiens, 2) the echogenic approximated mucosal surfaces of the outer bowel wall and the thicker, hypoechoic external returning limb of the intussusceptum, 3) the approximated echogenic serosal surfaces of the walls of the entering and returning limbs of the intussusceptum, 4) a variable amount of echogenic, eccentric mesentery with its associated vessels and lymph nodes pulled along with the entering limb, and 5) the central hypoechoic entering limb of the intussusceptum.

This semilunar, hyperechoic, mesenteric fat pulled into the center of the mass, the crescent-in-doughnut sign (**Fig. 23**), has been purported to be a characteristic feature of intussusception, enabling its sonographic differentiation from other types of GI disease.[76] In the absence of edema and mucosal breakdown, the sequential layers of the serosa, muscle, mucosa, muscle, and mesenteric fat create multiple concentric rings or an onion skin appearance (**Fig. 24**).[76,81] As the intussusception becomes more congested and edematous, however, it becomes more difficult to identify the individual layers.

When scanning through the longitudinal axis of the intussusception, the sonographic appearance varies with the appearance of the mesentery.[69] At the apex of the intussusception, thin strips of mesentery separate the three hypoechoic bowel loops, producing the hayfork sign (**Fig. 25**). In the midintussusception, there are outer hypoechoic bands consisting of the intussuscipiens and thickened everted limb of the intussusceptum separated from the central hypoechoic limb of the intussusception by entrapped mesentery, creating the sandwich sign (**Fig. 26**). If the intussusception is scanned slightly obliquely, only one side of the echogenic mesentery is seen along the central limb creating the pseudokidney sign (**Fig. 27**).

Ultrasound is also useful in identifying the presence of an underlying pathologic lead point (PLP), reported in 1.5% to 12% of children with intussusception.[65] The most common lead points are Meckel diverticulum, duplication cyst, polyp, and lymphoma. Although age over 5 years often is

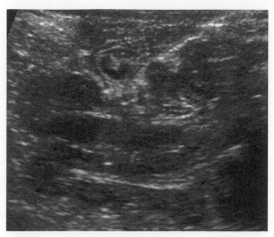

Fig. 25. Intussusception, hayfork sign. Longitudinal image of the leading edge of the intussusception demonstrating the hayfork sign.

cited as a predictor of the presence of a PLP (60% in 5- to 14-year age group), most intussusceptions caused by pathologic lead points occur in the first year of life.[66,67,82,83] Other clinical clues include an underlying disease known to predispose to intussusception like a polyposis syndrome, cystic fibrosis, or Henoch-Schonlein purpura; a history of recurrent intussusceptions; and atypical location of the intussusceptions.[82] Sonography has been shown to detect approximately two thirds of PLPs and enable the specific diagnosis of approximately one third. Ultrasound is particularly helpful in the diagnosis of lymphoma, which appears as a lobulated hypoechoic mass (**Fig. 28**) and duplication cyst

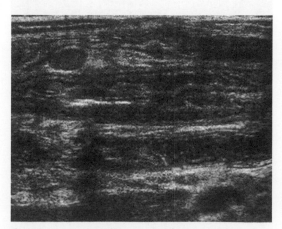

Fig. 26. Intussusception, sandwich sign. Longitudinal image demonstrates the layers of intussusception forming the sandwich sign.

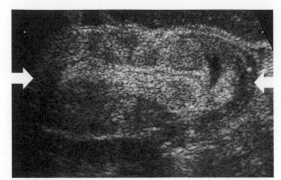

Fig. 27. Intussusception, pseudokidney sign. Longitudinal image through one aspect of the intussuscepted mesentery producing the pseudokidney sign (*between arrows*).

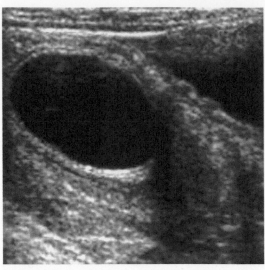

Fig. 29. Intussusception, pathologic lead point. Ileal duplication cyst at the leading edge of an intussusception.

(**Fig. 29**), but less so in the cases of Meckel diverticulum, which presents as a bulbous, elongated, or teardrop-shaped mass with a thickened wall surrounding fat (**Fig. 30**) and polyps (**Fig. 31**).[65]

Several sonographic features have been suggested as potential predictors of irreducibility by enema. Some have argued that the target appearance with multiple concentric rings is reducible due to little or no vascular compromise, while the thickened (>10 mm) hypoechoic outer rim of the doughnut sign is a manifestation of bowel edema and ischemia, and therefore is less reducible.[72,84] The data on thickness, however, are inconclusive.[76,77,84,85] Initially, it was thought that color Doppler sonography might differentiate viable from gangrenous bowel in intussusception.

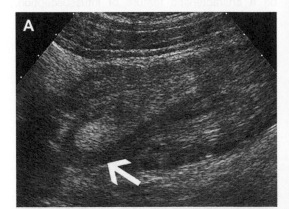

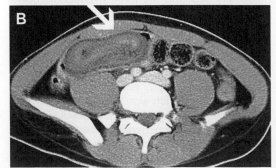

Fig. 30. Meckel diverticulum as PLP for intussusception. (*A*) A blind-ending, thick-walled inverted Meckel diverticulum surrounding echogenic fat (*arrow*) is the PLP for an intussusception in a 16-year-old boy with abdominal pain and Down syndrome. (*B*) Corresponding CT image showing intussusception (*arrow*).

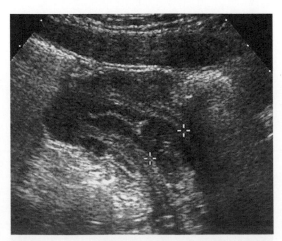

Fig. 28. Intussusception, pathologic lead point. Transverse RLQ image shows an appendix thickened by lymphoma (*cursors*) acting as a pathologic lead point for intussusception.

Subsequent studies have demonstrated a lower reduction rate of those intussusceptions without color Doppler signal, but up to a third without detectable flow remained reducible.[86] The presence of trapped peritoneal fluid within the intussusceptum, particularly if the fluid is greater than 8 × 3 mm and located at the apex, is associated with lower reported reduction rates of 25% to 26% (**Fig. 32**),[84,87] as compared with the expected successful reduction rate of approximately 80%.[67] The presence of at least two enlarged lymph nodes, one of which is greater than 11 mm in the intussusception, also has been reported to decrease the subsequent reduction rate (46%) (**Fig. 33**).[88] Finally, intussusceptions secondary to pathologic lead points are associated with slightly decreased reducibility (50% to 60%).[82] Although none of the preceding sonographic features precludes a reduction attempt, a recent article documents a significant risk of bowel necrosis and perforation with the presence of intramural or subserosal gas, manifested as echogenic foci, within the intussusception on ultrasound.[89] Therefore, in the presence of intramural or subserosal gas, one should proceed to reduction with extreme caution.

In contrast to the idiopathic intussusception, intussusceptions confined to the small bowel are usually small, transient, idiopathic, and asymptomatic, and involve a short segment of bowel in the central or left side of the abdomen (**Fig. 34**).[65] They are often incidental findings on cross-sectional imaging performed for other reasons. The sonographic features are similar to those of idiopathic intussusceptions.[90,91] Persistent, symptomatic small bowel intussusceptions may require surgical intervention. Although rarely identified prospectively with ultrasound,

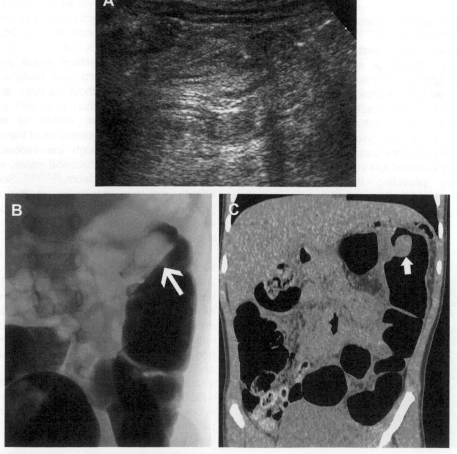

Fig. 31. Juvenile polyp causing colo-colonic intussusception. (*A*) Transverse sonographic image of a juvenile polyp located at the splenic flexure producing a colo-colonic intussusception in a 4-year-old child. (*B*) Diagnostic water-soluble enema demonstrating the polyp (*arrow*). (*C*) Noncontrasted coronal CT image demonstrating the colonic polyp (*arrow*).

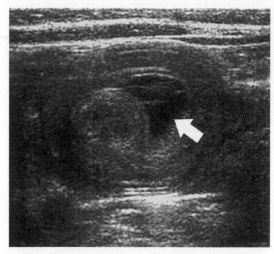

Fig. 32. Intussusception, entrapped fluid. Transverse sonographic image of an intussusception shows entrapped interloop fluid (*arrow*) and thickened wall at the apex of an intussusception, suggesting decreased reducibility.

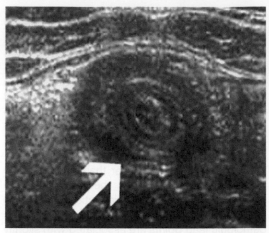

Fig. 34. Small bowel intussusception. Small bowel intussusceptions (*arrow*) are typically transient, smaller, and more centrally located than ileocolic intussusceptions.

pathologic lead points often are found at operation (42% to 69% of cases).[66,90] In small bowel intussusceptions, length greater than 3.5 cm has been shown to be a sensitive and specific predictor of the need for surgical intervention.[90]

Various reduction techniques have been developed to treat intussusception. They all use a combination of a contrast agent (fluid or air) under direct imaging guidance (fluoroscopy or sonography). In some parts of the world, sonography plays a central role in the treatment of intussusception, providing the primary imaging guidance for both hydrostatic and pneumatic reductions.

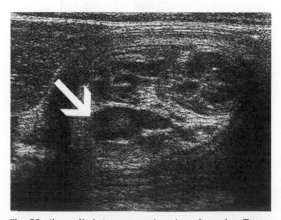

Fig. 33. Ileocolic intussusception, lymph nodes. Transverse sonographic image shows an ileocolic intussusception containing several enlarged lymph nodes (*arrow*) trapped within the mesentery.

Ultrasound-guided hydrostatic reductions have been shown to have reduction rates comparable to those of other methods, (67% to 95.5%) with few complications (2.7% to 4.26%) (**Fig. 35**).[92–102] Proponents of this method argue that in the absence of radiation exposure, multiple attempts may be performed without concern, and risk of perforation is lower than that with pneumatic reduction. Sonographic criteria of successful reduction include disappearance of the characteristic target sign through the ileocecal valve, demonstration of the ileocecal valve, and reflux of fluid into the distal ileum.[39,98–100] Sonography affords real-time monitoring of the reduction process, potential identification of pathologic lead points, recognition of perforation or the presence of residual intussusception.

In Asia, sonography has been used in combination with rectal insufflation of air with reported success rates of 92% to 95%.[103–105] Those who have performed this technique report that even though air typically blocks effective ultrasound, in pneumatic reduction, the air remains distal to the intussusception and does not hinder the identification of the mass.[103] Intermittent scanning of the epigastrium is necessary to look for free intraperitoneal air as evidenced by ring down artifact in the subphrenic region.[105] Sonographic criteria for successful pneumatic reduction include the disappearance of the concentric rings of intussusception and identification of an abrupt transition between swollen terminal ileum and more proximal normal ileal loops on longitudinal scanning.[104,105] Although this method seems to combine the most effective contrast media with the least

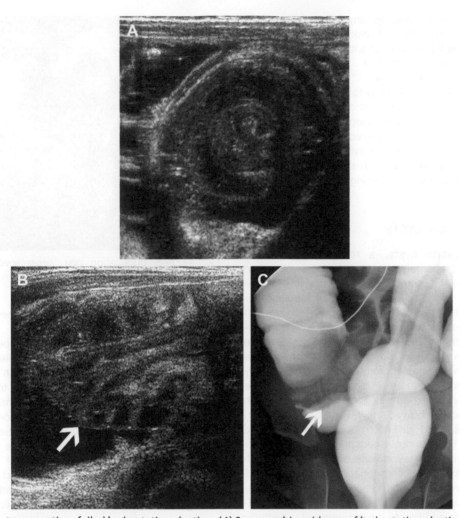

Fig. 35. Intussusception, failed hydrostatic reduction. (*A*) Sonographic guidance of hydrostatic reduction of intussusception using water-soluble contrast. The column of contrast is just reaching the apex of the intussusception. (*B*) Sonographic guidance of hydrostatic intussusception reduction demonstrating residual intussusception (*arrow*) extending through the ileocecal valve. (*C*) Synchronous fluoroscopic image demonstrates the residual intussusception (*arrow*) in the cecum.

harmful imaging modality, to date, it has failed to gain widespread acceptance.

The clear advantage of sonographic guidance of intussusception reduction is the lack of radiation exposure to the patient. Despite the exhortations to image gently, fluoroscopically guided reduction techniques still predominate in North America.[106,107] Proponents of fluoroscopy argue that sonographic guidance is more difficult, time-consuming, and messy and requires multiple individuals. Others fear an inability to recognize a reduction-induced perforation.[66,106] For many, choice of reduction technique boils down to a level of comfort.

Nonetheless, sonography still plays a pivotal role in fluoroscopically guided reduction techniques. Ultrasound is very effective in the confirmation of reduction or identification of residual ileoileal intussusception. It is particularly useful: 1) When pneumatic reduction is equivocal, as in the case of the disappearance of the intussusception from the colon but failure of air to reflux freely into small bowel; 2) In those patients with a small bowel obstruction and distended air-filled small bowel loops hindering those patients with a small bowel obstruction and distended air-filled small bowel loops hindering the ability to appreciate reflux of air into the terminal ileum.[108]

Sonography also has a role in the differentiation of a markedly thickened ileocecal valve from residual intussusception or potential lead point seen on air enema. In any of the previously mentioned scenarios, if residual intussusception is identified by ultrasound and the patient remains clinically stable, repeat delayed reduction attempts may be pursued.[109–111] Similarly, sonography is the ideal modality to evaluate the patient with recurrent or persistent abdominal pain after initial successful intussusception reduction.[64,108] It affords identification of a recurrence of the intussusception or alternatively evidence of an ongoing inflammatory process such as mesenteric adenopathy, bowel wall thickening, and hyperemia.[110]

DUPLICATION CYSTS

GI duplication cysts, a relatively uncommon congenital anomaly, may occur in any location along the GI tract and may be multiple in number.[112,113] They are spherical or tubular fluid-filled cysts lined by intestinal epithelium and an outer muscular wall, and they are closely approximated with a portion of the GI tract (**Fig. 36**). More than 50% occur in the small intestine, with the ileum being the most common site.[114] They usually are found within the mesentery and share a common blood supply and muscular wall with the adjacent bowel; however, they maintain a separate and distinct mucosal lining.[112] The intestinal lining is not necessarily that of the adjacent bowel but may include ectopic tissue such as gastric (43% of esophageal, 24% of small bowel, and 29% of thoracoabdominal duplications) or pancreatic mucosa (37% of gastric duplications). In addition to the presence of potentially clinically significant ectopic tissue, enteric duplication cysts may be associated with atresias (9%) and vertebral anomalies.[112] Duplication cysts may present at any age, but most present during infancy. Several are identified by prenatal ultrasound and referred for postnatal evaluation.[115] Postnatally, the clinical presentation is variable but includes abdominal pain, obstruction, bleeding, and a palpable abdominal mass. Pain may result from distension or rupture of the cyst, peptic ulceration, pancreatitis, bowel obstruction, or intussusception.[112]

Ultrasound plays a vital role in the diagnosis of intra-abdominal enteric duplications. Sonography not only readily identifies the cyst and its anatomic location, but also the hallmark gut signature of its wall, a 1 mm to 2 mm, fuzzy, echogenic inner rim of mucosa surrounded by a 1 mm to 2 mm sonolucent outer layer of muscularis (**Fig. 37**). The double layers are evident in more than 50% of the cysts and are better delineated in the far wall of the cyst.[116] Use of a high-frequency linear

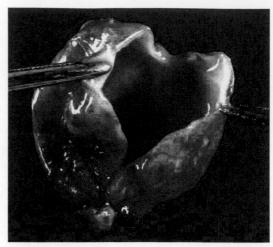

Fig. 36. Ileal duplication cyst. Gross specimen of a surgically resected ileal duplication cyst.

transducer will enable detailed assessment of the cyst wall.

Careful sonographic technique is important to identify potential mimics of the double-layered wall. An interface artifact may produce a focal, sharp, double-wall sign localized to the most dependent portion of other abdominal cysts, which disappears with slight angulation of the transducer.[116] Other reported potential sonographic mimics of duplication cysts include torsion of an ovarian cyst or Meckel diverticulum,[117,118] cystic ovarian tumors, and mesenteric cysts.[119] It would be very difficult to distinguish a torsed Meckel diverticulum from

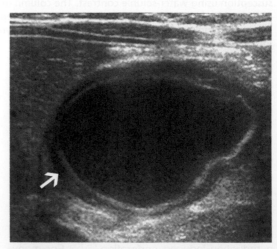

Fig. 37. Gastric duplication cyst. Transverse sonographic image shows a gastric duplication cyst demonstrating the characteristic double-layered wall with echogenic mucosa and hypoechoic muscular wall (*arrow*).

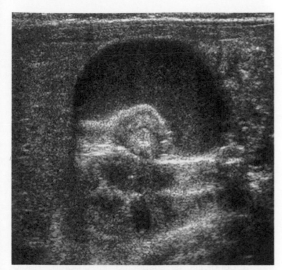

Fig. 38. Cecal duplication cyst. Sagittal sonographic image of a cecal duplication cyst with internal debris in a newborn.

a duplication cyst, as they both have the characteristic sonographic gut signature. Any other cyst with an inner echogenic lining comprised of fat, calcium, or epithelium and an outer hypoechoic fibrous wall could produce a pseudogut signature and cause a false-positive diagnosis of duplication cyst. Furthermore, not all duplication cysts are simple cysts. The internal character of an enteric cyst may be complicated by hemorrhage, inspissated mucous, or infectious debris (**Fig. 38**). In a case of an infected duplication cyst, the inner lining may ulcerate and erode, thereby destroying the characteristic inner echogenic layer and obscuring the correct diagnosis.[119] Notwithstanding these potential pitfalls, the presence of a cyst with a double-layered wall is highly suggestive of an enteric duplication. Sonographic observation of peristalsis within the wall and the presence of five sonographic layers (superficial and deep mucosa, submucosa, muscularis propria, and serosa) provide added specificity to the diagnosis.[120,121]

SUMMARY

Ultrasound is an outstanding tool in the evaluation of the child with acute abdominal pain, affording the diagnosis of appendicitis, intussusception, and duplication cyst with a high degree of accuracy. It may be helpful in providing alternative diagnoses such as omental infarction or mesenteric adenitis. Sonography can confirm clinically suspected pancreatitis and identify potential complications. Identification of bowel wall thickening may suggest gastroenteritis or colitis in the appropriate clinical setting, IBD if the symptoms are

more chronic, HSP if there is an associated purpuric rash, or lymphoma if the thickening is marked and associated with an abdominal mass. In addition to providing valuable diagnostic information, ultrasound can be performed readily in the acute setting with little or no patient preparation and without the risk of radiation exposure.

REFERENCES

1. Patino MO, Munden MM. Utility of the sonographic whirlpool sign in diagnosing midgut volvulus in patients with atypical clinical presentations. J Ultrasound Med 2004;23:397–401.
2. Jayaraman MV, Mayo-Smith WW, Movson JS, et al. CT of the duodenum: an overlooked segment gets its due. Radiographics 2001;21:S147–60.
3. Yousefzadeh D. The position of the duodenojejunal junction: the wrong horse to bet on in diagnosing or excluding malrotation. Pediatr Radiol 2009; 39(Suppl 2):S172–7.
4. Spechler SJ, Schimmel EM, Kressel HY. Serum amylase in pancreatitis. Dig Dis Sci 2005;30:92–3.
5. Benifla M, Weizman Z. Acute pancreatitis in childhood: analysis of literature data. J Clin Gastroenterol 2003;37:169–72.
6. Kovanlikaya A, Mittelman SD, Ward A, et al. Obesity and fat quantification in lean tissues using three-point Dixon MR imaging. Pediatr Radiol 2005; 35:601–7.
7. Bluth EI, Benson CB, Ralls PW, et al, editors. Ultrasound: a practical approach to clinical problems. New York: Thieme; 2007.
8. Chao HC, Lin SJ, Kong MS, et al. Sonographic evaluation of the pancreatic duct in normal children and children with pancreatitis. J Ultrasound Med 2000;19:757–63.
9. Andronikou S, Sinclair-Smith C, Millar AJ. An enteric duplication cyst of the pancreas causing abdominal pain and pancreatitis in a child. Pediatr Surg Int 2002;18:190–2.
10. Ozel A, Uysal E, Tufaner O, et al. Duodenal duplication cyst: a rare cause of acute pancreatitis in children. J Clin Ultrasound 2008;36:584–6.
11. Bjerring OS, Durup J, Qvist N, et al. Impact of upper gastrointestinal endoscopic ultrasound in children. J Pediatr Gastroenterol Nutr 2008;47: 110–3.
12. Varadarajulu S, Wilcox CM, Eloubeidi MA. Impact of EUS in the evaluation of pancreaticobiliary disorders in children. Gastrointest Endosc 2005;62: 239–44.
13. Addiss DG, Shaffer N, Fowler BS, et al. The epidemiology of appendicitis and appendectomy in the United States. Am J Epidemiol 1990;132:910–25.

14. Rothrock SG, Pagane J. Acute appendicitis in children: emergency department diagnosis and management. Ann Emerg Med 2000;36:39–51.

15. Sivit CJ, Newman KD, Boenning DA, et al. Appendicitis: usefulness of US in diagnosis in a pediatric population. Radiology 1992;185:549–52.

16. Jorwitz JF, Gursoy M, Jaksic T, et al. Importance of diarrhea as a presenting symptom of appendicitis in very young children. Am J Surg 1997;173:80–2.

17. Williams N, Bello M. Perforation rate relates to delayed presentation in childhood acute appendicitis. J R Coll Surg Edinb 1998;43:101–2.

18. Rodriguez DP, Vargas S, Callahan MJ, et al. Appendicitis in young children: imaging experience and clinical outcomes. AJR Am J Roentgenol 2006;186:1158–64.

19. Rothrock SG, Skeoch G, Rush JJ, et al. Clinical features of misdiagnosed appendicitis in children. Ann Emerg Med 1991;20:45–50.

20. Puylaert JB. Acute appendicitis: US evaluation using graded compression. Radiology 1986;158:355–60.

21. Lee JH, Jeong YK, Park KB, et al. Operator-dependent techniques for graded compression sonography to detect the appendix and diagnose acute appendicitis. AJR Am J Roentgenol 2005;184:91–7.

22. Baldisserotto M, Marchiori E. Accuracy of noncompressive sonography of children with appendicitis according to the potential positions of the appendix. AJR Am J Roentgenol 2000;175:1387–92.

23. Wiersma F, Sramek A, Holscher HC. US features of the normal appendix and surrounding area in children. Radiology 2005;235:1018–22.

24. Jeffrey RB, Jain KA, Nghiem HV. Sonographic diagnosis of acute appendicitis: interpretive pitfalls. AJR Am J Roentgenol 1994;162:55–9.

25. Lim HK, Lee WJ, Lee SJ, et al. Focal appendicitis confined to the tip: diagnosis at US. Radiology 1996;200:799–801.

26. Lim HK, Lee WJ, Kim TH, et al. Appendicitis: usefulness of color Doppler US. Radiology 1996;201:221–5.

27. Lee MW, Kim YJ, Jeon HJ, et al. Sonography of acute right lower quadrant pain: importance of increased intraabdominal fat echo. AJR Am J Roentgenol 2009;192:174–9.

28. Noguchi T, Yoshimitsu K, Yoshida M. Periappendiceal hyperechoic structure on sonography: a sign of severe appendicitis. J Ultrasound Med 2005;24:323–7 [quiz: 328–30].

29. Himeno S, Yasuda S, Oida Y, et al. Ultrasonography for the diagnosis of acute appendicitis. Tokai J Exp Clin Med 2003;28:39–44.

30. Wiersma F, Toorenvliet BR, Bloem JL, et al. US examination of the appendix in children with suspected appendicitis: the additional value of secondary signs. Eur Radiol 2009;19:455–61.

31. Levin T, Whyte C, Borzykowski R, et al. Nonoperative management of perforated appendicitis in children: can CT predict outcome? Pediatr Radiol 2007;37:251–5.

32. Whyte C, Levin T, Harris BH. Early decisions in perforated appendicitis in children: lessons from a study of nonoperative management. J Pediatr Surg 2008;43:1459–63.

33. Menten R, Lebecque P, Saint-Martin C, et al. Outer diameter of the vermiform appendix: not a valid sonographic criterion for acute appendicitis in patients with cystic fibrosis. AJR Am J Roentgenol 2005;184:1901–3.

34. Kao CT, Tsai JD, Lee HC, et al. Right perinephric abscess: a rare presentation of ruptured retrocecal appendicitis. Pediatr Nephrol 2002;17:177–80.

35. Sivit CJ, Siegel MJ, Applegate KE, et al. When appendicitis is suspected in children. Radiographics 2001;21:247–62 [questionnaire 288–94].

36. Macari M, Hines J, Balthazar E, et al. Mesenteric adenitis: CT diagnosis of primary versus secondary causes, incidence, and clinical significance in pediatric and adult patients. AJR Am J Roentgenol 2002;178:853–8.

37. Rao PM, Rhea JT, Novelline RA. CT diagnosis of mesenteric adenitis. Radiology 1997;202:145–9.

38. Rao R, Lowas S, Shashidhar H. Surgical complications of Salmonella Enteritis. Clin Pediatr (Phila) 2005;44:767–9.

39. Haber HP, Busch A, Ziebach R, et al. Ultrasonographic findings correspond to clinical, endoscopic, and histologic findings in inflammatory bowel disease and other enterocolitides. J Ultrasound Med 2002;21:375–82.

40. Matsumoto T, Iida M, Sakai T, et al. Yersinia terminal ileitis: sonographic findings in eight patients. AJR Am J Roentgenol 1991;156:965–7.

41. van Breda Vriesman AC, Puylaert JB. Mimics of appendicitis: alternative nonsurgical diagnoses with sonography and CT. AJR Am J Roentgenol 2006;186:1103–12.

42. d'Almeida M, Jose J, Oneto J, Restrepo R. Bowel wall thickening in children: CT findings. Radiographics 2008;28:727–46.

43. Miller FH, Ma JJ, Scholz FJ. Imaging features of enterohemorrhagic Escherichia coli colitis. AJR Am J Roentgenol 2001;177:619–23.

44. Tanaka O, Matsuura K, Nagai J, et al. Hemorrhagic colitis caused by Escherichia coli preceding hemolytic–uremic syndrome: radiologic features. AJR Am J Roentgenol 1992;158:551–2.

45. Ledermann HP, Borner N, Strunk H, et al. Bowel wall thickening on transabdominal sonography. AJR Am J Roentgenol 2000;174:107–17.

46. Lim JH, Ko YT, Lee DH, et al. Sonography of inflammatory bowel disease: findings and value in differential diagnosis. AJR Am J Roentgenol 1994;163:343–7.

47. O'Malley ME, Wilson SR. US of gastrointestinal tract abnormalities with CT correlation. Radiographics 2003;23(1):59–72.

48. Sturm EJ, Cobben LP, Meijssen MA, et al. Detection of ileocecal Crohn's disease using ultrasound as the primary imaging modality. Eur Radiol 2004; 14:778–82.

49. Ripolles T, Martinez MJ, Morote V, et al. Appendiceal involvement in Crohn's disease: gray-scale sonography and color Doppler flow features. AJR Am J Roentgenol 2006;186:1071–8.

50. Puylaert JB. Right-sided segmental infarction of the omentum: clinical, US, and CT findings. Radiology 1992;185:169–72.

51. Baldisserotto M, Maffazzoni DR, Dora MD. Omental infarction in children: color Doppler sonography correlated with surgery and pathology findings. AJR Am J Roentgenol 2005;184:156–62.

52. van Breda Vriesman AC, Puylaert JB. Omental infarction: a self-limiting disease. AJR Am J Roentgenol 2005;185:280 [author reply 280–1].

53. Grattan-Smith JD, Blews DE, Brand T. Omental infarction in pediatric patients: sonographic and CT findings. AJR Am J Roentgenol 2002;178:1537–9.

54. Surawicz CM, McFarland LV. Pseudomembranous colitis: causes and cures. Digestion 1999;60: 91–100.

55. Downey DB, Wilson SR. Pseudomembranous colitis: sonographic features. Radiology 1991;180:61–4.

56. Russo P, Brown K, Baldassano RN. In: Russo P, Ruchelli E, Piccoli DA, editors. Pathology of pediatric gastrointestinal and liver disease. New York (NY): Springer; 2004. Chapter 5.

57. Johnson PT, Horton KM, Fishman EK. Case 127: henoch-schonlein purpura. Radiology 2007;245: 909–13.

58. Macari M, Chandarana H, Balthazar E, et al. Intestinal ischemia versus intramural hemorrhage: CT evaluation. AJR Am J Roentgenol 2003;180:177–84.

59. John S, Swischuk E, Hayden CK, et al. Gastrointestinal sonographic findings in Henoch-Schonlein purpura. Emergency Radiol 1996;3:4–8.

60. Levine MS, Rubesin SE, Pantongrag-Brown L, et al. Non-Hodgkin's lymphoma of the gastrointestinal tract: radiographic findings. AJR Am J Roentgenol 1997;168:165–72.

61. Ferry JA. Burkitt's lymphoma: clinicopathologic features and differential diagnosis. Oncologist 2006;11:375–83.

62. Toma P, Granata C, Rossi A, et al. Multimodality imaging of Hodgkin disease and non-Hodgkin lymphomas in children. Radiographics 2007;27: 1335–54.

63. Parashar UD, Holman RC, Cummings KC, et al. Trends in intussusception-associated hospitalizations and deaths among US infants. Pediatrics 2000;106:1413–21.

64. Applegate KE. Intussusception in children: evidence-based diagnosis and treatment. Pediatr Radiol 2009;39(Suppl 2):S140–3.

65. Navarro O, Daneman A. Intussusception. Part 3: diagnosis and management of those with an identifiable or predisposing cause and those that reduce spontaneously. Pediatr Radiol 2004;34: 305–12 [quiz: 369].

66. Ko HS, Schenk JP, Troger J, et al. Current radiological management of intussusception in children. Eur Radiol 2007;17:2411–21.

67. Daneman A, Navarro O. Intussusception. Part 1: a review of diagnostic approaches. Pediatr Radiol 2003;33:79–85.

68. Harrington L, Connolly B, Hu X, et al. Ultrasonographic and clinical predictors of intussusception. J Pediatr 1998;132:836–9.

69. del-Pozo G, Albillos JC, Tejedor D, et al. Intussusception in children: current concepts in diagnosis and enema reduction. Radiographics 1999;19:299–319.

70. Applegate KE. Clinically suspected intussusception in children: evidence-based review and self-assessment module. AJR Am J Roentgenol 2005; 185:S175–83.

71. Schmit P, Rohrschneider WK, Christmann D. Intestinal intussusception survey about diagnostic and nonsurgical therapeutic procedures. Pediatr Radiol 1999;29:752–61.

72. Swischuk LE, Hayden CK, Boulden T. Intussusception: indications for ultrasonography and an explanation of the doughnut and pseudokidney signs. Pediatr Radiol 1985;15:388–91.

73. Eshed I, Gorenstein A, Serour F, et al. Intussusception in children: can we rely on screening sonography performed by junior residents? Pediatr Radiol 2004;34:134–7.

74. Henrikson S, Blane CE, Koujok K, et al. The effect of screening sonography on the positive rate of enemas for intussusception. Pediatr Radiol 2003; 33:190–3.

75. Lim HK, Bae SH, Lee KH, et al. Assessment of reducibility of ileocolic intussusception in children: usefulness of color Doppler sonography. Radiology 1994;191:781–5.

76. del-Pozo G, Albillos JC, Tejedor D. Intussusception: US findings with pathologic correlation—the crescent-in-doughnut sign. Radiology 1996;199: 688–92.

77. Verschelden P, Filiatrault D, Garel L, et al. Intussusception in children: reliability of US in diagnosis—a prospective study. Radiology 1992;184:741–4.

78. Alessi V, Salerno G. The hay-fork sign in the ultrasonographic diagnosis of intussusception. Gastrointest Radiol 1985;10:177–9.

79. Bowerman RA, Silver TM, Jaffe MH. Real-time ultrasound diagnosis of intussusception in children. Radiology 1982;143:527–9.

80. Friedman AP, Haller JO, Schneider M, et al. The pediatric corner. Sonographic appearance of intussusception in children. Am J Gastroenterol 1979;72:92–4.

81. Holt S, Samuel E. Multiple concentric ring sign in the ultrasonographic diagnosis of intussusception. Gastrointest Radiol 1978;3:307–9.

82. Navarro O, Dugougeat F, Kornecki A, et al. The impact of imaging in the management of intussusception owing to pathologic lead points in children. A review of 43 cases. Pediatr Radiol 2000;30: 594–603.

83. Ong NT, Beasley SW. The leadpoint in intussusception. J Pediatr Surg 1990;25:640–3.

84. Britton I, Wilkinson AG. Ultrasound features of intussusception predicting outcome of air enema. Pediatr Radiol 1999;29:705–10.

85. Mirilas P, Koumanidou C, Vakaki M, et al. Sonographic features indicative of hydrostatic reducibility of intestinal intussusception in infancy and early childhood. Eur Radiol 2001;11:2576–80.

86. Kong MS, Wong HF, Lin SL, et al. Factors related to detection of blood flow by color Doppler ultrasonography in intussusception. J Ultrasound Med 1997;16:141–4.

87. del-Pozo G, Gonzalez-Spinola J, Gomez-Anson B, et al. Intussusception: trapped peritoneal fluid detected with US—relationship to reducibility and ischemia. Radiology 1996;201:379–83.

88. Koumanidou C, Vakaki M, Pitsoulakis G, et al. Sonographic detection of lymph nodes in the intussusception of infants and young children: clinical evaluation and hydrostatic reduction. AJR Am J Roentgenol 2002;178:445–50.

89. Stranzinger E, Dipietro MA, Yarram S, et al. Intramural and subserosal echogenic foci on US in large-bowel intussusceptions: prognostic indicator for reducibility? Pediatr Radiol 2009;39:42–6.

90. Munden MM, Bruzzi JF, Coley BD, et al. Sonography of pediatric small-bowel intussusception: differentiating surgical from nonsurgical cases. AJR Am J Roentgenol 2007;188:275–9.

91. Tiao MM, Wan YL, Ng SH, et al. Sonographic features of small-bowel intussusception in pediatric patients. Acad Emerg Med 2001;8:368–73.

92. Bai YZ, Qu RB, Wang GD, et al. Ultrasound-guided hydrostatic reduction of intussusceptions by saline enema: a review of 5218 cases in 17 years. Am J Surg 2006;192:273–5.

93. Choi SO, Park WH, Woo SK. Ultrasound-guided water enema: an alternative method of nonoperative treatment for childhood intussusception. J Pediatr Surg 1994;29:498–500.

94. Crystal P, Hertzanu Y, Farber B, et al. Sonographically guided hydrostatic reduction of intussusception in children. J Clin Ultrasound 2002;30:343–8.

95. del Pozo G. Intussusception: still work in progress. Pediatr Radiol 2005;35:92–4 [author reply 95–6].

96. Gonzalez-Spinola J, Del Pozo G, Tejedor D, et al. Intussusception: the accuracy of ultrasound-guided saline enema and the usefulness of a delayed attempt at reduction. J Pediatr Surg 1999; 34:1016–20.

97. Hadidi AT, El Shal N. Childhood intussusception: a comparative study of nonsurgical management. J Pediatr Surg 1999;34:304–7.

98. Peh WC, Khong PL, Chan KL, et al. Sonographically guided hydrostatic reduction of childhood intussusception using Hartmann's solution. AJR Am J Roentgenol 1996;167:1237–41.

99. Riebel TW, Nasir R, Weber K. US-guided hydrostatic reduction of intussusception in children. Radiology 1993;188:513–6.

100. Rohrschneider WK, Troger J. Hydrostatic reduction of intussusception under US guidance. Pediatr Radiol 1995;25:530–4.

101. Wang GD, Liu SJ. Enema reduction of intussusception by hydrostatic pressure under ultrasound guidance: a report of 377 cases. J Pediatr Surg 1988; 23:814–8.

102. Wood SK, Kim JS, Suh SJ, et al. Childhood intussusception: US-guided hydrostatic reduction. Radiology 1992;182:77–80.

103. Gu L, Zhu H, Wang S, et al. Sonographic guidance of air enema for intussusception reduction in children. Pediatr Radiol 2000;30:339–42.

104. Lee JH, Choi SH, Jeong YK, et al. Intermittent sonographic guidance in air enemas for reduction of childhood intussusception. J Ultrasound Med 2006;25:1125–30.

105. Yoon CH, Kim HJ, Goo HW. Intussusception in children: US-guided pneumatic reduction—initial experience. Radiology 2001;218:85–8.

106. Daneman A, Navarro O. Intussusception: the debate endures. Pediatr Radiol 2005;35:95–6.

107. Khanna G, Applegate K. Ultrasound-guided intussusception reduction: are we there yet? Abdom Imaging 2008;33:38–40.

108. Daneman A, Navarro O. Intussusception. Part 2: an update on the evolution of management. Pediatr Radiol 2004;34:97–108 [quiz: 187].

109. Connolly B, Alton DJ, Ein SH, et al. Partially reduced intussusception: when are repeated delayed reduction attempts appropriate? Pediatr Radiol 1995;25:104–7.

110. Navarro OM, Daneman A, Chae A. Intussusception: the use of delayed, repeated reduction attempts and the management of intussusceptions due to pathologic lead points in pediatric patients. AJR Am J Roentgenol 2004;182: 1169–76.

111. Sandler AD, Ein SH, Connolly B, et al. Unsuccessful air-enema reduction of intussusception: is a second attempt worthwhile? Pediatr Surg Int 1999;15:214–6.

112. Macpherson RI. Gastrointestinal tract duplications: clinical, pathologic, etiologic, and radiologic considerations. Radiographics 1993;13:1063–80.

113. Sutcliffe J, Munden M. Sonographic diagnosis of multiple gastric duplication cysts causing gastric outlet obstruction in a pediatric patient. J Ultrasound Med 2006;25:1223–6.

114. Hur J, Yoon CS, Kim MJ, et al. Imaging features of gastrointestinal tract duplications in infants and children: from oesophagus to rectum. Pediatr Radiol 2007;37:691–9.

115. Khong PL, Cheung SC, Leong LL, et al. Ultrasonography of intra-abdominal cystic lesions in the newborn. Clin Radiol 2003;58:449–54.

116. Barr LL, Hayden CK Jr, Stansberry SD, et al. Enteric duplication cysts in children: are their ultrasonographic wall characteristics diagnostic? Pediatr Radiol 1990;20:326–8.

117. Gallego-Herrero C, del Pozo-Garcia G, Marin-Rodriguez C, et al. Torsion of a Meckel's diverticulum: sonographic findings. Pediatr Radiol 1998;28:599–601.

118. Godfrey H, Abernethy L, Boothroyd A. Torsion of an ovarian cyst mimicking enteric duplication cyst on transabdominal ultrasound: two cases. Pediatr Radiol 1998;28:171–3.

119. Cheng G, Soboleski D, Daneman A, et al. Sonographic pitfalls in the diagnosis of enteric duplication cysts. AJR Am J Roentgenol 2005;184:521–5.

120. Simonovsky V. Jejunal duplication cyst displaying peristalsis and a five-layered appearance of the wall: a preoperative ultrasound diagnosis. Eur Radiol 1996;6:153–5.

121. Spottswood SE. Peristalsis in duplication cyst: a new diagnostic sonographic finding. Pediatr Radiol 1994;24:344–5.

Ultrasound of Pediatric Liver Masses

Laura Varich, MD[a,b]

KEYWORDS

- Liver tumor • Pediatric • Ultrasound

This article provides an overview of the ultrasound (US) imaging of liver masses. The first section covers general concepts of hepatic mass evaluation by US. The second section is devoted to a more detailed discussion of each tumor type. Where applicable, specific tumor presentations are followed by "key diagnostic points," which summarize the important differentiating features of each lesion.

GENERAL CONCEPTS

The liver is embryologically derived from both mesenchymal and endodermal tissues and can, therefore, develop a wide variety of both benign and malignant neoplasms.[1] Primary hepatic neoplasms are the third most common abdominal malignancy in childhood, after Wilms tumor and neuroblastoma, and two-thirds of pediatric hepatic tumors are malignant. US has an important role as the first-line imaging technique for hepatic masses in children based on the modality's safety and accessibility. The main goals of imaging are to (1) define the organ of origin, (2) determine the tumor type where possible, (3) delineate potential surgical resectability, and (4) assess response to therapy.

Defining the Organ of Origin

Pediatric abdominal masses are often very large at presentation; thus, defining the organ of origin can be difficult, as hepatic masses may be confused with primary renal or adrenal tumors.

The real-time and multiplanar capability of US, as well as the modality's exquisite evaluation of vascular structures, can provide helpful clues to the hepatic origin of a mass by defining any of the following: a hepatic artery feeding the mass, enlargement of the hepatic artery (signifying intratumoral vascular shunting), displacement or invasion of the segmental portal veins or hepatic veins, and movement of the mass with the liver during respiration.[2]

Determining Tumor Type

Although a hepatic mass in a child may occasionally have a characteristic appearance, in most cases the tumor type cannot be diagnosed with certainty via imaging. Therefore, the clinical presentation, patient age at diagnosis, alphafetoprotein (AFP) level, number of hepatic lesions, vascular characteristics of the lesion, and presence of normal or abnormal underlying liver parenchyma are frequently pieces of information essential to narrowing the differential diagnostic considerations.

In most patients with either benign or malignant hepatic masses, the clinical presentation is a palpable mass on physical examination. These patients may or may not present with additional signs and/or symptoms, such as pain, jaundice, hemorrhage, and congestive heart failure. Congestive heart failure is most frequently associated with infantile hepatic hemangiomas owing to significant intratumoral arteriovenous shunting.

It is critical to consider the age of the patient when formulating a differential diagnosis list for pediatric liver tumors given that the tumor types encountered vary significantly with patient age. In patients younger than 5 years, benign infantile hemangioma, mesenchymal hamartoma, hepatoblastoma, and metastatic disease from neuroblastoma, leukemia, and Wilms tumor are the most common hepatic neoplasms encountered. In patients older than 5 years, the most common

---

[a] Florida Hospital for Children, 601 East Rollins Street, Orlando, FL 32803, USA
[b] Stanford University Medical Center, Stanford, CA, USA
E-mail address: laura.varich@gmail.com

Ultrasound Clin 5 (2010) 137–152
doi:10.1016/j.cult.2009.11.011

masses are hepatocellular carcinoma, undifferentiated embryonal sarcoma, hepatic adenoma, metastatic disease, lymphoma, and focal nodular hyperplasia.

Serum protein levels may be of benefit in the diagnosis of hepatic masses. For example, AFP levels are elevated in 90% of patients harboring hepatoblastoma and in 50% to 75% of patients with hepatocellular carcinoma. AFP is only rarely elevated in infantile hemangiomas. Thus, AFP is a very useful diagnostic tool, as an elevated AFP level strongly suggests hepatoblastoma or hepatocellular carcinoma in patients younger or older than 5 years, respectively. Similarly, urine protein levels may be of diagnostic benefit. Urine catecholamine levels are elevated in more than 90% of patients suffering from neuroblastoma.[3]

The number of hepatic lesions also guides the diagnosis. Multiplicity of hepatic masses favors the diagnosis of metastatic disease, benign infantile hemangioma, lymphoproliferative disease, or adenomas related to an underlying metabolic syndrome.

Vascular characteristics of a liver mass are also meaningful and can be evaluated by Doppler imaging and, where available, the newer technique of contrast-enhanced US. In liver masses, benign and malignant lesions can demonstrate differing Doppler patterns. Studies have demonstrated that malignant lesions tend to display an elevated systolic Doppler shift of greater than 2.5 kHz[4] or 4 kHz[5]; however, this finding overlaps with results demonstrated in benign infantile hemangiomas.[6] Most benign lesions tend to have no increase in systolic Doppler shift.[4,5]

US contrast agents serve to increase US signal. Differing agents and techniques can be useful for increasing conspicuity of hepatic lesions by altering their signal compared with background, for evaluating lesion vascularity and dynamic enhancement characteristics, and for appraising the vascular characteristics of tumors by assessing perfusion and washout characteristics seen at early and delayed imaging. Contrast-enhanced US is not yet available for routine use in the United States. Clinical use of this technology in other countries has demonstrated a potential to improve visualization and characterization of liver masses,[2,7,8] and experience with this technique continues to grow. Evaluation of lesion vascularity has reported the following characteristics: hepatocellular carcinoma has linear but dysmorphic vessels, focal nodular hyperplasia has linear and stellate vascularity, and infantile hemangiomas have peripheral puddling.[7] Imaging with contrast in the portal venous phase has demonstrated utility in differentiating benign and malignant

primary liver masses. Both benign and malignant lesions tend to demonstrate increased echogenicity in the arterial phase compared with background liver (indicating hepatic arterial supply). The portal venous phase, though, has been found to demonstrate early washout (and, therefore, hypoechogenicity) in malignant lesions (including metastases) and sustained vascularity (persistent increased echogenicity) in benign lesions.[7,8]

The Doppler and contrast-enhanced US findings are not yet specific enough to be used as isolated diagnostic tools but should be included when possible in the overall diagnostic process when evaluating the potential benign or malignant nature of a hepatic lesion.

In children with liver masses, the underlying liver parenchyma can demonstrate evidence of chronic liver disease, with implications for the lesions that occur in this setting. In pediatric patients, the two most common such scenarios are hepatocellular carcinoma, presenting within a background of cirrhosis, and hepatic adenomas, where depositional diseases cause the liver to appear enlarged and echogenic.

Delineating Potential Surgical Resectability

The staging of primary malignant liver tumors in children is heavily dependent upon delineation of intrahepatic tumor spread and, therefore, US plays a key role in tumor staging. Two main systems are currently used for the staging of primary malignant liver tumors in children. In North America, the Intergroup Staging System is most often used. The Intergroup Staging System is largely dependent upon the outcome of attempted surgical resection.[9] Thus, preoperative US plays a key role in determining likelihood of success and approach to liver resection. In many other countries, the PRETEXT (pretreatment extent of disease) system is used. This system is based in large part on the extent of the intrahepatic tumor spread as delineated by preoperative imaging, including US.[10-12]

Thus, in either staging system, the extent of tumor involvement within the liver and the surgical resectability are crucial to staging. In cases of suspected malignancy, the radiologist must identify the number of hepatic lesions, the segments of liver involved, any involvement of the portal and hepatic venous systems and inferior vena cava, and the presence of extrahepatic spread. Venous involvement by tumor is indicative of malignancy (particularly hepatocellular carcinoma) and more often suggestive of a primary, rather than metastatic, tumor. When vascular flow is identified within a thrombus or enlargement of the occluded vein is seen, malignant thrombus should be suspected. When evaluating the hepatic segmental anatomy, the Couinaud system is most commonly used.[13] Using this classification, conventional liver resection (including hemihepatectomy and extended hemihepatectomy) can be performed if tumor involvement spares at least the left lateral segment of the liver (segments 2 and 3) or the lateral segments of the right lobe of the liver (segments 6 and 7). US is a valuable tool in evaluation of resectability, as US allows real-time evaluation of the tumor in relation to the hepatic vasculature.[14]

Evidence of extrahepatic spread, such as lymph node metastasis or direct tumor spread to adjacent organs or the peritoneum, should also be sought. The presence of extrahepatic spread will advance the tumor stage, potentially affecting therapeutic options. The subtleties of extrahepatic spread relative to tumor type must be appreciated. For example, extrahepatic spread of tumor is very rare in cases of hepatoblastoma.[11] Extrahepatic extension of tumor should be differentiated from the relatively common exophytic or pedunculated tumor growth pattern in hepatoblastoma. This type of growth is considered confined to the liver if no invasion of adjacent structures is noted.[11] Invasion into local structures may be more common with hepatocellular carcinoma, as 10% of adult patients are noted to have diaphragmatic invasion by tumor.[11] Peritoneal spread and tumor rupture can be demonstrated by US in both hepatocellular carcinoma and hepatoblastoma. Peritoneal spread of malignancy can be seen in the presence of ascites, where nodular implants are visualized along the peritoneal surfaces. Tumor rupture is suggested by discontinuity of the tumor margin and the presence of echogenic material within the ascitic fluid, whereas subcapsular hemorrhage does not imply tumor rupture.[11]

Patients with malignant disease who are deemed surgically unresectable, even those with involvement of the hepatic vasculature or inferior vena cava, may be candidates for liver transplantation. Excellent results for primary liver transplantation have been demonstrated in patients with hepatoblastoma, with a 6-year survival rate of 82% after primary orthotopic liver transplantation.[15] Even patients suffering from a primary liver tumor with metastatic spread may qualify for transplantation if the metastases are successfully treated by pretransplantation chemotherapy or surgical resection.[14]

Assessment of Response to Therapy

Depending on the tumor type and extent of hepatic involvement, patients may receive chemotherapy,

radiation, surgical resection, liver transplantation, or a combination of these therapies. US is an excellent tool for evaluating hepatic tumor therapeutic response. Critical to determining therapeutic responsiveness of hepatic lesions is consistency in imaging parameters and technique, allowing for accurate measurement of changes in tumor mass.

PRIMARY BENIGN HEPATIC NEOPLASMS
Benign Infantile Hemangioma (Hemangioendothelioma)

Infantile hemangioma is the most common hepatic neoplasm of infancy[16] and the most common benign hepatic tumor of childhood.[17] Infantile hemangioma is an endothelial cell neoplasm with an early proliferative phase associated with rapid growth. This phase occurs in the first 6 months to 2 years of life and can be associated with increased vascularity and significant arteriovenous shunting. The lesion then undergoes spontaneous involution, a phase that lasts months to years. By adolescence, most infantile hemangiomas have undergone complete regression. The nomenclature used for vascular lesions is often confusing, and the lesion described here has also been called hemangioendothelioma or infantile hepatic hemangioma. No matter which terminology is used, the nomenclature attempts to differentiate this benign infantile lesion from 2 noninvoluting lesions: the epithelioid hemangioendothelioma, a proliferative lesion that possesses malignant potential, and the adult hepatic hemangioma, thought to represent a venous vascular malformation.[18]

The vast majority of patients with benign infantile hemangiomas present before 6 months of age.[1] Presenting signs and symptoms include congestive heart failure (related to vascular shunting), hepatomegaly, anemia, jaundice, and coagulopathy (related to platelet sequestration, the Kasabach-Merritt syndrome). This lesion can be identified even in the fetus using prenatal US by identification of a liver mass of variable echogenicity with increased flow on Doppler US, cardiac compromise, and hydrops.[1] Approximately half of patients with benign infantile hemangioma of the liver have associated cutaneous hemangiomas, thought to be part of a diffuse process of hemangiomatosis.[19,20]

In patients with a typical presentation and imaging findings, the diagnosis of infantile hemangioma may be made by US imaging alone. On US, these lesions are most often multifocal; however, they can also present as solitary or diffuse.[18] The multifocal infantile hemangiomas often appear as numerous, small, well-defined, hypoechoic lesions that can involve a single hepatic segment or the entire liver (**Fig. 1**). Infrequently, the multifocal masses can appear hyperechoic. Solitary lesions are usually larger and may become heterogeneous in appearance as a result of central hemorrhage or necrosis. In the diffuse type of benign infantile hemangioma, the liver may appear enlarged and heterogeneous without discrete identifiable lesions. All imaging patterns of benign infantile hemangioma may demonstrate finely speckled internal calcifications. Infantile hemangiomas are classically noted to have multiple, large, tortuous vessels within the lesion and at the periphery (**Fig. 2**). Doppler interrogation demonstrates elevated Doppler shifts compared with normal hepatic vessels.[6] If there is a significant degree of arteriovenous shunting, there may be enlargement of the celiac artery and hepatic artery, along with decrease in the caliber of the infra-celiac aorta (**Fig. 3**). This finding is characteristic of infantile hemangioma but may be noted in other types of tumors in which significant arteriovenous shunting is present. Doppler US may also identify enlargement of the draining hepatic veins (**Fig. 4**), which can appear "arterialized" with increased pulsatility and flow velocity.[21]

In patients whose presentation or imaging findings are atypical, a definitive diagnosis of infantile hemangioma may be difficult to make. Imaging findings in cases of infantile hemangioma are not always specific, as there is significant crossover between the appearance of hemangioma and other benign and malignant lesions. If signs of hypervascularity (such as enlarged vessels on gray-

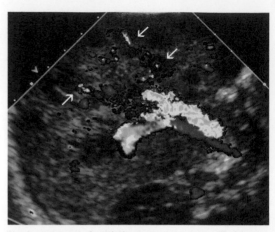

Fig. 2. Benign infantile hemangioma. Transverse color Doppler sonogram (same patient as **Fig. 1**) demonstrates hypervascularity within and around the nodules (*arrows*). Enlarged hepatic arteries and portal veins also noted centrally at the porta hepatis.

scale imaging) are not identified, infantile hemangioma may be indistinguishable from other neoplasms,[18] and even the appearance of hypervascularity is not specific enough to confidently differentiate infantile hemangioma from hypervascular malignancies (**Fig. 5**). An abnormal Doppler shift pattern seen in infantile hemangiomas[6] is also not on its own a reliable diagnostic finding, as this same pattern may be seen in malignant lesions.[2] In atypical imaging cases, the vascular nature of the mass can be confirmed by bolus contrast injection and multiphase computed tomography (CT) or magnetic resonance (MR) imaging. Infantile hemangiomas will be seen to

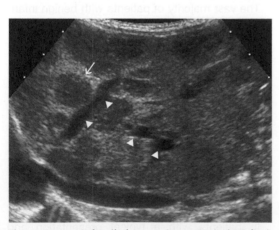

Fig. 1. Benign infantile hemangioma. Typical US findings in an infant with an enlarged liver. Sagittal sonogram illustrates the classic appearance of infantile hemangioma of the liver with multiple hypoechoic nodules (one indicated by an arrow) and enlarged hepatic vessels (*arrowheads*).

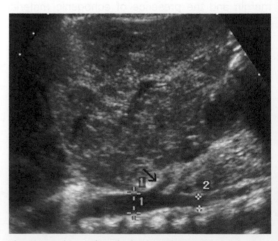

Fig. 3. Benign infantile hemangioma. Sagittal sonogram of the aorta reveals abrupt tapering of the aorta below the celiac axis owing to significant arteriovenous shunting. Cursors delineate diameter of the aorta above and below the celiac artery (*arrow*).

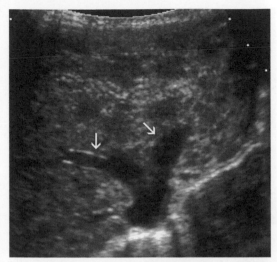

Fig. 4. Benign infantile hemangioma. Transverse sonogram demonstrates enlarged hepatic veins (*arrows*) secondary to arteriovenous shunting. Also note the numerous hypoechoic liver nodules.

enhance homogeneously or in centripetal fashion, with the lesion enhancing peripherally in the early phase and progressing to fill in centrally on later phases[18] (**Fig. 6**). This pattern of contrast enhancement on CT or MR imaging is highly correlated with infantile hemangioma. A similar pattern of enhancement has been reported with contrast-enhanced US.[7] Rare cases have been reported of an identical pattern of contrast enhancement in cases of hypervascular hepatoblastoma,[22,23] although AFP levels should be elevated in these patients. Large solitary infantile

hemangiomas may lack the classic central enhancement pattern because of central necrosis.

The natural history of infantile hemangioma is gradual involution and cessation of clinical symptoms. The prognosis in affected children is dependent upon the clinical status of the patient. Asymptomatic patients diagnosed incidentally do very well, whereas a poorer prognosis is associated with patients suffering severe, life-threatening congestive heart failure or platelet sequestration. In this latter patient population, therapy including steroids and alpha-interferon, angiography and vascular embolization, surgical resection, and even liver transplantation has been advocated[24] in an attempt to improve survival. Malignant transformation of this lesion into angiosarcoma has been reported but is rare.[20,25]

Key diagnostic points

Benign infantile hemangioma of the liver may demonstrate a variable gray-scale appearance but most often consists of multifocal hypoechoic nodules. Key US findings include enlarged feeding, draining, and intralesional vessels demonstrating increased systolic Doppler shift and peripheral puddling of contrast on early post–contrast-enhanced US, CT, or MR imaging.

Mesenchymal Hamartoma

Mesenchymal hamartoma is the second most common benign liver tumor in children, usually identified within the first 2 years of life. This lesion is believed to be a developmental anomaly of the portal connective tissue rather than a true neoplasm and is composed of both mesenchymal

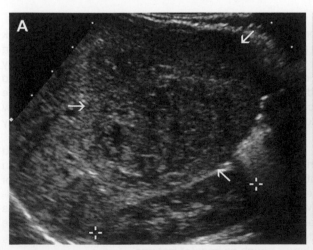
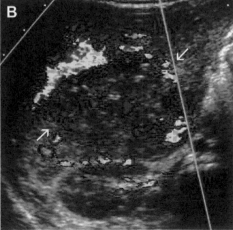

Fig. 5. Benign infantile hemangioma in a 4-month-old with a palpable abdominal mass. (*A*) Sagittal gray-scale sonogram of the liver depicts a solitary focal liver mass (*arrows*) without distinguishing characteristics. (*B*) Transverse sonogram of the mass with color Doppler demonstrates hypervascularity (*arrows*), a nonspecific finding that can be seen in other hypervascular tumors.

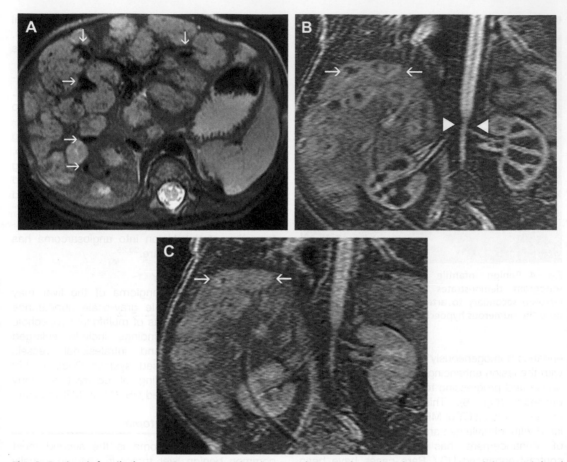

Fig. 6. Benign infantile hemangioma presenting in a newborn evaluated with MR imaging. (*A*) T2-weighted image shows multiple hyperintense nodules and hypervascularity as demonstrated by large flow voids (*arrows*). (*B*) Coronal T1-weighted image in the arterial phase of contrast enhancement demonstrates peripheral enhancement of the hepatic lesions (2 such lesions are indicated by arrows). Significant tapering of the aorta below the celiac axis is also evident (*arrowheads*). (*C*) Coronal T1-weighted image in a delayed phase of enhancement reveals central filling in of the lesions (the same 2 lesions are indicated by arrows).

and epithelial components. Cystic degeneration of the mesenchyme with fluid accumulation from obstructed lymphatics or bile ducts produces the classic cystic appearance of the lesion and can lead to rapid enlargement of the tumor.[26] Children harboring a mesenchymal hamartoma typically present with an asymptomatic, enlarging abdominal mass.

At imaging, classic findings of the lesion are those of a large mass most often involving the right lobe of the liver, with a cystic and multiseptate appearance. These masses are usually large at diagnosis, with 85% of patients presenting with masses measuring greater than 10 cm in one published series.[27] US imaging may demonstrate 3 different appearances: a well-defined, solitary lesion that appears cystic and multiseptate; a mixed cystic and solid lesion ("Swiss-cheese appearance"); or, less commonly, a completely

solid lesion (**Fig. 7**). Septations may be thin or thick and can even be associated with nodularity. On US, solid components of the lesion are usually heterogeneous and iso- to slightly hyperechoic to liver.[27] The solid tissue and septations within the lesion often demonstrate low-level vascular flow on Doppler imaging. The cyst contents may appear anechoic or may contain debris.

The gray-scale imaging characteristics in mixed cystic and solid lesions may overlap with benign infantile hemangioma; however, in the case of mesenchymal hamartoma, no increased vascularity is seen on color Doppler US. In patients with solid tumors, the imaging characteristics are not specific enough to exclude malignant lesions, such as hepatoblastoma.

There have been a few reports of malignant degeneration of mesenchymal hamartoma, particularly into undifferentiated embryonal sarcoma,[28–30]

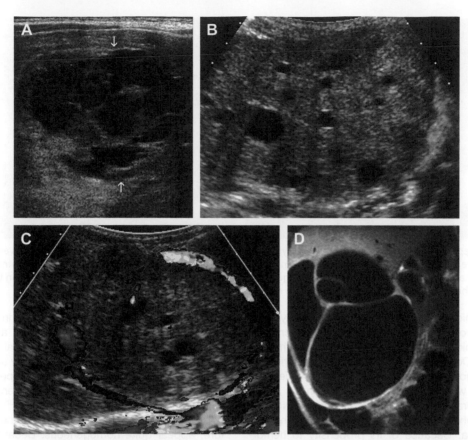

Fig. 7. Mesenchymal hamartoma of the liver in 3 infants. (*A*) Transverse sonogram of the liver reveals a multicystic mass (*arrows*) with thick septations. (*B*) Transverse sonogram demonstrates a mixed cystic and solid liver mass involving most of the visualized segment of liver with a "Swiss-cheese appearance." (*C*) Color Doppler imaging of the same mass in **Fig. 7b** shows hypovascularity and displacement of the hepatic vessels. (*D*) Coronal T1-weighted MR image demonstrates a very large multicystic liver mass with thin septations.

but as surgical resection is the standard treatment for mesenchymal hamartoma,[31] the potential for malignant degeneration is avoided, and the patient is provided with an excellent long-term prognosis.

Key diagnostic points
Mesenchymal hamartoma should be the primary diagnostic consideration for a cystic mass identified within the liver of a child younger than 2 years.

Hepatic Adenoma

Hepatic adenoma is a rare lesion in children. When it occurs, it is usually found in association with metabolic disease (particularly glycogen storage disease), anabolic steroid therapy for Fanconi anemia, or oral contraceptive therapy. Hepatic adenomas are composed of cords of hepatocytes demonstrating increased intracellular fat and glycogen and separated by dilated, thin-walled, vascular sinusoids. These thin-walled sinusoids are fed by hepatic arteries and, therefore, perfused

at arterial pressures, resulting in a propensity to hemorrhage.[32] These lesions are also reported to possess an increased risk of malignant degeneration into hepatocellular carcinoma.[33]

Hepatic adenomas may be detected in patients during screening for the previously mentioned predisposing conditions. Patients with or without an underlying condition may present with hepatic enlargement, right upper quadrant discomfort, and/or severe abdominal pain secondary to tumor hemorrhage or rupture.

US imaging may demonstrate multiple masses (particularly in patients with predisposing conditions) or a solitary mass. Individual adenomas may vary from 1 cm to greater than 15 cm in size[32] and appear round and sharply marginated. US characteristics are not specific, as lesions may vary from hyper- to hypoechoic[2] and hyper- to hypovascular (**Fig. 8**).[34] The presence of internal fat or calcification (related to areas of necrosis) may produce focal areas of increased

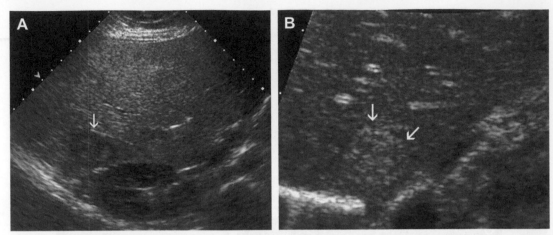

Fig. 8. Hepatic adenoma in 2 patients. (*A*) A 5-year-old girl with Type 1 glycogen storage disease. Transverse sonogram reveals a small mixed-echogenicity lesion (*arrow*) within the right lobe of the liver. The underlying liver is enlarged and echogenic consistent with glycogen storage disease. (*B*) A hyperechoic mass is identified in the right lobe of the liver (*arrows*) in a teenage girl on oral contraceptive therapy.

echogenicity. Intratumoral hemorrhage may result in heterogeneity and increased or decreased echogenicity, depending on the age of the hemorrhage. Doppler US will demonstrate peripheral peri-tumoral feeding vessels and intralesional vessels with continuous flow or triphasic flow[32] and midrange Doppler shifts (2–4 kHz).[2] None of these sonographic findings are specific for hepatic adenoma. Because of its propensity to hemorrhage, rupture, or undergo malignant degeneration, differentiation of hepatic adenomas from other benign and malignant hepatic tumors is critical. Therefore, many of these patients also undergo MR or CT imaging, where characteristic findings may be identified.[32]

The prognosis in hepatic adenoma patients is not clear. Hepatic adenomas may regress or may increase in size over time. Given the risk of hemorrhage and malignant degeneration, surgical excision is usually performed after initial diagnosis.

Key diagnostic points
The US imaging findings of hepatic adenoma are nonspecific. Multiple hepatic lesions in a child who has one of the predisposing conditions are suggestive of this diagnosis.

Focal Nodular Hyperplasia
Focal nodular hyperplasia (FNH) is most often diagnosed in middle-aged women and is a rare finding in children. FNH is a benign tumor that likely represents a hyperplastic response of hepatocytes to a congenital vascular anomaly.[35] FNH lesions are often asymptomatic and found incidentally. Symptomatic patients may complain of an abdominal mass or abdominal pain.

FNH is usually a solitary lesion measuring smaller than 5 cm that appears lobulated and well defined. It has a characteristic central fibrotic scar with feeding arteries noted centrally and radiating along fibrous septa to the periphery. Because FNH lesions have an excellent blood supply and do not grow to a large size,[35] they do not undergo hemorrhage or necrosis and, therefore, appear quite homogeneous. Because FNH is composed of hyperplastic but otherwise normal hepatocytes, the lesion most often appears isoechoic to slightly hypoechoic to liver and can be difficult to visualize on US (**Fig. 9**). Some FNH lesions may be detected only by their displacement of vessels or by visualization of the central scar. If the central scar is identified, it appears hyperechoic, and the central artery may be visualized by color Doppler. If the characteristic findings are noted on US, a prospective diagnosis may be made. More often, additional imaging is required, with MR being the imaging choice related to its improved sensitivity and specificity and lack of ionizing radiation. MR imaging will demonstrate a mass that has similar signal intensity to normal liver. The central scar is vascularized and demonstrates high T2 signal intensity.[36]

FNH is a benign lesion without malignant potential. Therefore, no treatment or follow-up is required in asymptomatic patients who present with classic imaging findings. If the diagnosis is not certain after imaging and malignant lesions remain in the differential diagnosis, subsequent imaging, biopsy, or surgical resection may be indicated.

Key diagnostic points
The characteristic findings of FNH include a hepatic lesion that is relatively small (smaller

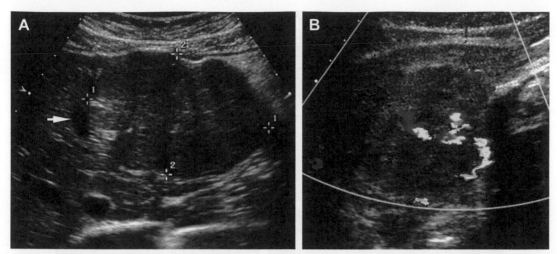

Fig. 9. Focal nodular hyperplasia in a 12-year-old boy. (*A*) Transverse sonogram shows a lobular mass (*cursors*) in the left hepatic lobe that is nearly isoechoic to the adjacent liver and displaces the left hepatic vein (*arrow*). (*B*) Longitudinal color Doppler image shows a central feeding artery. (*Courtesy of* Brian D. Coley, MD, Columbus, OH.)

than 5 cm) and nearly isoechoic to normal liver parenchyma, with a hyperechoic central scar that demonstrates central vasculature with a stellate arrangement of vessels flowing to the periphery. Other imaging patterns seen in FNH are nonspecific, and the lesion may require additional imaging with MR for diagnosis.

PRIMARY MALIGNANT HEPATIC NEOPLASMS
Hepatoblastoma

Hepatoblastoma is the most common primary malignancy of the liver in childhood. Hepatoblastoma is usually diagnosed in infants and children younger than 3 years and has even been diagnosed prenatally.[1] This tumor most often is composed solely of epithelial cells, either of the fetal type (the most favorable histology), embryonal type, or mixed fetal and embryonal type. Less commonly, hepatoblastoma is composed of mixed epithelial and mesenchymal cells (the least favorable histology).[19] This less-favorable subtype often has differentiated osteoid tissue identified at pathologic analysis, which appears as coarse or chunky calcification on imaging.[37] Increased incidence of hepatoblastoma is noted in association with Beckwith-Weidemann syndrome, hemihypertrophy, low birth weight, and familial adenomatous polyposis. Cirrhosis is not a risk factor. Patients with hepatoblastoma are usually asymptomatic and are found to have hepatomegaly or a large liver mass on physical examination. Serum AFP level is elevated in more than 90% of patients.

Hepatoblastoma is most often a large solitary mass that is located within the right lobe of the liver. Less common patterns include multinodularity and diffuse liver involvement. Calcification may be noted and often corresponds with the unfavorable lesion of mixed histology.[37] On US imaging, the mass is usually heterogeneous and hyperechoic to normal liver parenchyma and has ill-defined margins (**Fig. 10**). The remaining liver appears normal. Internal hypoechoic or anechoic areas often represent foci of hemorrhage or necrosis. Hepatoblastoma is a hypervascular mass (**Fig. 11**). Doppler evaluation of vessels will demonstrate elevated peak systolic Doppler frequency shifts (<4 kHz) consistent with arteriovenous shunting and associated with malignant neovascularity.[5]

Treatment of hepatoblastoma includes surgical resection and chemotherapy. The goal of therapy is complete surgical resection, without which cure is rare. Surgical resectability depends on the number of segments and vessels involved, and is best determined with MR imaging[2]; 50% to 60% of tumors are found to be resectable at diagnosis. In the remainder, preoperative chemotherapy is required to decrease the tumor to resectable size. The overall survival after treatment for hepatoblastoma is 60% to 70%, correlating with those patients who undergo successful complete primary surgical resection. For patients who remain unresectable after preoperative chemotherapy, liver transplantation may be considered.

Key diagnostic points

Hepatoblastoma may have varied and nonspecific imaging findings; thus, the clinical presentation is

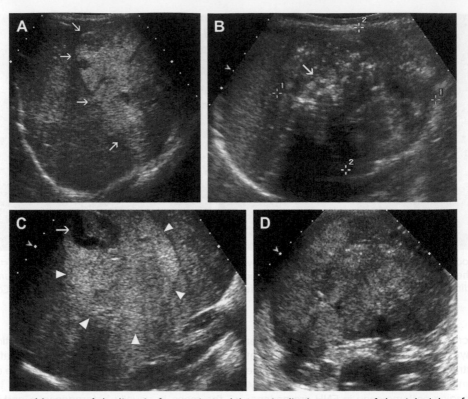

Fig. 10. Hepatoblastoma of the liver in four patients. (*A*) Longitudinal sonogram of the right lobe of the liver demonstrates a large lobulated hyperechoic mass (*arrows*). (*B*) Longitudinal sonogram reveals a heterogeneous focal mass (delineated by cursors) with course calcification (*arrow*) in the right lobe of the liver. (*C*) Longitudinal sonogram of the right lobe of the liver identifies a large heterogeneous hyperechoic mass (*arrowheads*) with anechoic foci of necrosis (*arrow*). (*D*) Transverse sonogram of the abdomen in an infant demonstrates a large diffusely infiltrating mass causing heterogeneity of the entire liver.

critical in aiding diagnosis. A hepatic mass presenting in a child younger than 3 years and with an elevated serum AFP level is almost always indicative of hepatoblastoma.

Hepatocellular Carcinoma

Hepatocellular carcinoma (HCC) is the second most common malignant hepatic neoplasm in children. HCC presents at an older age than does hepatoblastoma, with most HCC cases diagnosed in children older than 5 years. Up to 75% of patients will have elevated serum AFP levels.[38]

Patients most often present with an enlarging abdominal mass. The risk of HCC is elevated in patients suffering from chronic liver diseases, such as glycogen storage disease, cystinosis, tyrosinemia, Wilson disease, alpha1-antitrypsin deficiency, biliary cirrhosis related to biliary atresia, and posthepatitis cirrhosis.

HCC is a malignancy of hepatocyte origin. The tumor is noted to have a fibrous capsule and is also predisposed to vascular invasion. On US

imaging, HCC may appear as a solitary or multicentric mass most commonly involving the right lobe of the liver, or as a diffusely infiltrating lesion (**Fig. 12**). At diagnosis, these masses appear solid, rarely contain calcification, and have variable echogenicity. Small lesions appear homogeneous and are most often hypoechoic. The capsule can be seen as a hypoechoic halo. Larger lesions become necrotic, and therefore demonstrate a more heterogeneous appearance. Doppler US may detect the high-velocity flow that is related to neovascularity, but Doppler US is most useful for identifying venous invasion. Portal venous invasion is identified in up to 60% of cases,[2] with hepatic venous invasion identified less commonly (**Fig. 13**). Doppler US may differentiate neoplastic thrombus from bland (benign) thrombus by detecting internal neovascularity in the former.

The clinical presentation in patients suffering from HCC is often delayed until the tumor reaches a large size and an advanced stage; thus, unfortunately, only 15% to 30% of tumors are surgically resectable at diagnosis. Treatment of HCC differs is seen most often in young adults (age range of 5 to 35 years)[38] who present with pain, mass, fever, weight loss, and other constitutional symptoms. Serum AFP levels are normal. Because almost half of FLHCC tumors are resectable at diagnosis, these lesions are reportedly associated with a better prognosis than typical HCC (63% vs 30% 5-year survival),[39] although the authenticity of this reported difference has been debated.[40] FLHCC may demonstrate variable echogenicity, and calcification is present in 50% of cases.[38] A classic US finding in FLHCC is a central echogenic scar, noted in 60% of cases.[41] The central scar is a finding also seen in FNH but often can be differentiated by association of malignant characteristics (including ill definition and heterogeneity) and a low T1 and T2 signal intensity central scar that is poorly vascularized in FLHCC.[36] Surgical resection is usually performed after diagnosis of FLHCC.

Key diagnostic points

A liver mass in a child older than 5 years who also presents with an elevated serum AFP level should be considered HCC until otherwise proven.

Undifferentiated Embryonal Sarcoma

Undifferentiated embryonal sarcoma of the liver is a very rare, rapidly growing, and highly malignant tumor that occurs in older children and young adults. Serum AFP levels are normal. US imaging demonstrates a large, solitary, heterogeneous, echogenic mass with areas of internal necrosis or cystic degeneration.[42] The imaging characteristics are not specific, and clinical information (age and

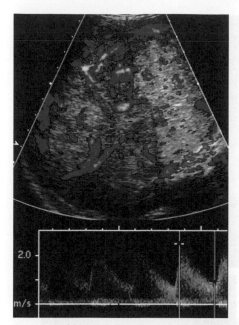

Fig. 11. Hepatoblastoma. Transverse power Doppler image in a 10-month-old shows a large heterogeneous liver mass with marked vascularity. Doppler waveform shows high-velocity low-resistance arterial flow. (*Courtesy of* Brian D. Coley, MD, Columbus, OH.)

from that of hepatoblastoma in that all patients undergo tumor resection at the time of diagnosis if possible, and preoperative chemotherapy is not usually administered.[14]

The fibrolamellar subtype of HCC (FLHCC) accounts for 3% of HCCs and is not associated with underlying liver disease. FLHCC lesions are solitary, encapsulated, and well defined. FLHCC

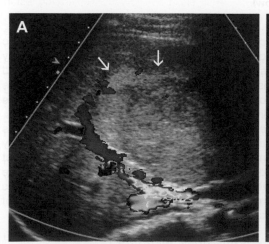
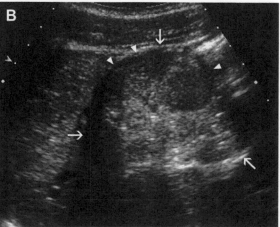

Fig. 12. Hepatocellular carcinoma, appearance in 2 patients. (*A*) Transverse color Doppler image of the liver shows a large focal heterogeneous mass (*arrows*) displacing the hepatic vessels in a patient with chronic hepatitis B. (*B*) Longitudinal sonogram of the liver demonstrates a large heterogeneous mass (*arrows*) involving the right lobe of the liver with a hypoechoic halo noted anteriorly (*arrowheads*).

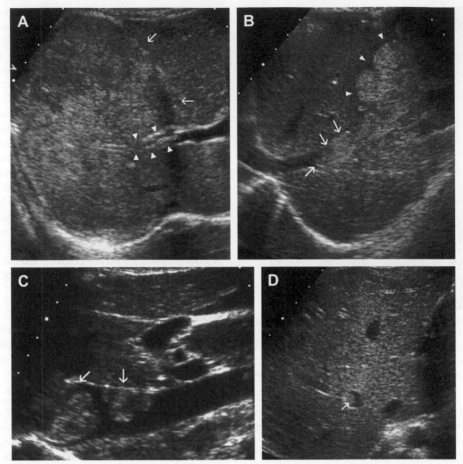

Fig. 13. Hepatocellular carcinoma with venous invasion in four patients. (*A*) Transverse sonogram of the liver demonstrates a large and infiltrative-appearing mass (*arrows*) involving the right lobe of the liver. The right portal vein is completely occluded with tumor thrombus (*arrowheads*). (*B*) Longitudinal sonogram reveals a large echogenic mass (*arrowheads*) with invasion of the inferior vena cava (IVC) (*arrows*). (*C*) Longitudinal sonogram of the liver in another patient with evidence of tumor thrombus in the IVC (*arrows*). (*D*) Transverse sonogram of the liver shows thrombus within the middle hepatic vein (*arrow*).

serum AFP level) may help differentiate this lesion from hepatoblastoma, HCC, and mesenchymal hamartoma. Prognosis for undifferentiated embryonal sarcoma patients is poor, with a median survival of 1 year.

Rhabdomyosarcoma of the Biliary Tract

Rhabdomyosarcoma of the biliary tract is a rare tumor that occurs in children with a mean age of 3.5 years.[2] US imaging findings may be suggestive if a lobulated intraluminal biliary mass can be identified in association with dilatation of the affected and obstructed biliary ducts.

SECONDARY NEOPLASMS OF THE LIVER

Secondary tumor involvement of the liver may be seen in metastatic disease and in patients with certain lymphoproliferative diseases. Metastatic disease of the liver in childhood is usually secondary to neuroblastoma or Wilms tumor and is most often identified as one or more nodules or masses of abnormal echogenicity within the liver parenchyma. In such metastatic cases, a complete abdominal US often demonstrates the adrenal, retroperitoneal, or renal primary malignancy. Lymphoproliferative diseases most often appear diffusely infiltrating when they involve the liver. A complete abdominal US in these cases may reveal lymphadenopathy or involvement of other organs.

Neuroblastoma Metastases

The liver is the most common site for neuroblastoma metastasis, and patients commonly present secondary to hepatic enlargement. More than

90% of patients with neuroblastoma have elevated urine catecholamines at diagnosis.[3] When the liver is evaluated sonographically, 2 metastatic patterns of involvement may be demonstrated: diffuse infiltration of the liver (more common in Stage IVS disease) and multiple nodules (Fig. 14).[1] Nodules may appear either hypo- or hyperechoic to normal liver parenchyma and may demonstrate variable vascularity. Stage IV and Stage IVS disease present with hepatic metastases; however, their course and prognoses are quite different. Patients with Stage IV disease have advanced tumor involvement including metastases to bone, liver, and/or lymph nodes. These patients are treated with aggressive chemotherapy and have a poor prognosis, with a 3-year survival of 15%.[43] Patients with Stage IVS disease present at younger than 1 year and have distant disease noted within the liver, skin, and bone marrow (not involving cortical bone). The natural history of Stage IVS disease is regression without treatment. These patients have an excellent prognosis, with a survival rate of greater than 90%.[43]

Wilms Tumor Metastases

In cases of Wilms tumor, the liver is the second most common site of metastasis after the lungs. Hepatic metastases are solitary or multiple, well defined, and of variable echogenicity[44] (Fig. 15). This tumor, even when metastatic, has an excellent prognosis, with a 4-year survival rate of 83% in patients suffering metastatic disease at the time of diagnosis.[43]

Lymphoproliferative Disease

Neoplastic hepatic involvement can also be seen in patients suffering from lymphoproliferative diseases, including leukemia or lymphoma, and in posttransplantation lymphoproliferative disorder. Patients in advanced stages of lymphoma often have secondary liver involvement. Extension of US imaging to include the entire abdomen will often demonstrate abnormal adenopathy or multiorgan involvement associated with lymphoma or leukemia. The most common pattern of hepatic metastatic involvement in these patients is diffuse

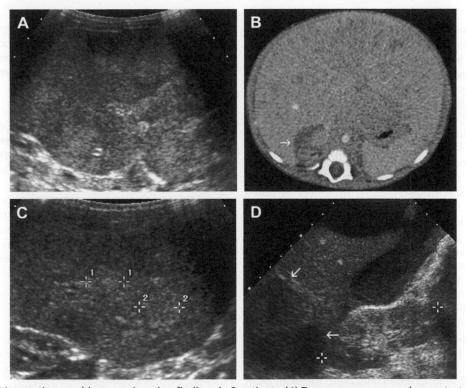

Fig. 14. Metastatic neuroblastoma, imaging findings in 3 patients. (A) Transverse sonogram demonstrates diffuse heterogeneity and enlargement of the liver in a patient with Stage IVS neuroblastoma. (B) Axial CT scan with contrast in the same patient as in Fig. 14A demonstrates the diffusely infiltrative appearance. The right adrenal primary tumor is also visualized (arrow). (C) Transverse-oblique sonogram depicts heterogeneity of the liver with multiple ill-defined hyperechoic lesions (marked by cursors) within the liver. (D) Longitudinal sonogram demonstrates a right adrenal primary lesion (arrows) and ascites in a patient with Stage IV disease (cursors mark the right kidney).

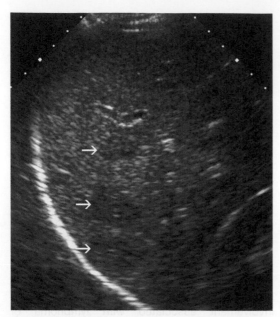

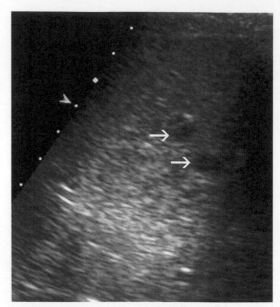

Fig. 15. Wilms tumor metastases. Longitudinal sonogram of the liver identifies at least 3 hypoechoic lesions of the liver (*arrows*), found to represent metastatic disease.

Fig. 16. Lymphoma with secondary liver involvement. On a background of liver enlargement and diffuse infiltration, 2 small anechoic appearing "cystlike" lesions (*arrows*) are seen.

infiltration of the hepatic parenchyma, and the only clue as to the presence of metastatic involvement may be liver enlargement. Occasionally, multiple homogeneous and hypoechoic nodules may be seen (**Fig. 16**). These nodules may appear so hypoechoic as to suggest cystic disease, but lack of posterior acoustic enhancement will clarify the solid nature of the masses.[45] If a single dominant mass is noted, it will appear larger and heterogeneous and more likely represents the rare case of primary lymphoma of the liver.

Posttransplantation lymphoproliferative disorder (PTLD) is a proliferation of B cells that occurs as early as 1 month to many years after solid organ or bone marrow transplantation. PTLD has an increased prevalence in children compared with adults (4.0% and 0.8%, respectively).[46] Immunosuppression causes decreased suppressor T-cell activity that results in a hyperproliferative response of B cells to Epstein-Barr virus (EBV) infection or reactivation. EBV initiates proliferation of a polyclonal cohort of lymphocytes, causing a masslike appearance in the transplanted organ or within other organs. If this polyclonal proliferation progresses unabated, transformation to a monoclonal line may occur, resembling lymphoma. In the liver, PTLD is often seen involving the lymphatic tissue along the portal triads. Findings may include hypoechoic thickening in the periportal soft tissues[47] or formation of discrete hypoechoic peripheral nodules, often

associated with the portal triads. Diagnosis of PTLD lesions requires biopsy. PTLD of a polyclonal cell type is treated by decreasing immunosuppression. Monoclonal PTLD behaves like lymphoma and is treated with chemotherapy.

Key diagnostic points
Diffuse infiltration of the liver is the most common presentation of metastatic spread to the liver in patients with leukemia and lymphoma. The presence of multiple masses within the liver is always suspicious for hepatic metastases or hepatic adenomas. A search for a potential primary malignant lesion (especially renal, adrenal, or retroperitoneal) should be performed. Thickening along the portal triads or multiple hypoechoic liver masses in a patient with a history of transplantation should raise suspicion for PTLD.

REFERENCES

1. Woodward PJ, Sohaey R, Kennedy A, et al. From the archives of the AFIP: a comprehensive review of fetal tumors with pathologic correlation. Radiographics 2005;25:215–42.
2. Rumack CM, Wilson SR, Charboneau JW. Diagnostic ultrasound. 3rd edition. St Louis (MO): Mosby; 2005.
3. Rivard DC, Lowe LH. Radiological reasoning: multiple hepatic masses in an infant. AJR Am J Roentgenol. 2008;190(Suppl 6):S46–52.

4. Van Campenhout I, Patriquin H. Malignant microvasculature in abdominal tumors in children: detection with Doppler US. Radiology 1992;183:445–8.

5. Bates SM, Keller MS, Ramos IM, et al. Hepatoblastoma: detection of tumor vascularity with duplex Doppler US. Radiology 1990;176(2):505–7.

6. Paltiel HJ, Patriquin HB, Keller MS, et al. Infantile hepatic hemangioma: Doppler US. Radiology 1992;182:735–42.

7. Brannigan M, Burns PN, Wilson SR. Blood flow patterns in focal liver lesions at microbubble-enhanced US. Radiographics 2004;24(4):921–35.

8. Jang HJ, Kim TK, Wilson SR. Imaging of malignant liver masses: characterization and detection. Ultrasound Q 2006;22(1):19–29.

9. Cohen MD, Bugaieski EM, Haliloglu M, et al. Visual presentation of the staging of pediatric solid tumors. Radiographics 1996;16:523–45.

10. Roebuck DJ, Aronson D, Clapuyt P, et al. 2005 PRETEXT: a revised staging system for primary malignant liver tumours of childhood developed by the SIOPEL group. Pediatr Radiol 2007;37:123–32.

11. Roebuck DJ, Sebire NJ, Pariente D. Assessment of extrahepatic abdominal extension in primary malignant liver tumours of childhood. Pediatr Radiol 2007;37:1096–100.

12. Roebuck DJ, Olsen O, Pariente D. Radiological staging in children with hepatoblastoma. Pediatr Radiol 2006;36:176–82.

13. Couinaud C. The paracaval segments of the liver. J Hepatobiliary Pancreat Surg 1994;2:145–51.

14. Czauderna P, Otte JB, Roebuck DJ, et al. Surgical treatment of hepatoblastoma in children. Pediatr Radiol 2006;36:187–91.

15. Otte JB, Aronson DC, Brown J, et al. Liver transplantation for hepatoblastoma. Results from the International Society of Pediatric Oncology (SIOP) study SIOPEL-1 and review of the world experience. Pediatr Blood Cancer 2004;42:74–83.

16. Chandra RS, Stocker JT. The liver, gallbladder, and biliary tract. In: Stocker JT, Dehner LP, editors. Pediatric pathology, vol. 2. Philadelphia: Lippincott; 1992.

17. Weinberg AG, Finegold MJ. Primary hepatic tumors of childhood. Hum Pathol 1983;14:512–37.

18. Kassarjian A, Zurakowski D, Dubois J, et al. Infantile hepatic hemangiomas: clinical and imaging findings and their correlation with therapy. AJR Am J Roentgenol 2004;182:785–95.

19. Kirks D. Practical pediatric imaging. 3rd edition. Philadelphia: Lippincott-Raven; 1998.

20. Keslar PJ, Buck JL, Selby DM. From the archives of the AFIP: infantile hemangioendothelioma of the liver revisited. Radiographics 1993;13:657–70.

21. Coley BD. Pediatric applications of abdominal vascular Doppler: part I. Pediatr Radiol. 2004; 34(10):757–71.

22. Lu M, Greer MC. Hypervascular multifocal hepatoblastoma: dynamic gadolinium-enhanced MRI findings indistinguishable from infantile hemangioendothelioma. Pediatr Radiol 2007;37:587–91.

23. Ingram DJ, Yerushalmi B, Connell J, et al. Hepatoblastoma in a neonate: a hypervascular presentation mimicking hemangioendothelioma. Pediatr Radiol 2000;30:794–7.

24. Kallcinski P, Ismall H, Broniszczak D, et al. Non-resectable hepatic tumors in children—role of liver transplantation. Ann Transplant 2008;13(2):37–41.

25. Kirchner SG, Heller RM, Kasselberg AG, et al. Infantile hepatic hemangioendothelioma with subsequent malignant degeneration. Pediatr Radiol 1981;11:42–5.

26. Stocker JT, Ishak KG. Mesenchymal hamartoma of the liver: report of 30 cases and review of the literature. Pediatr Pathol 1983;1:245–67.

27. Kim SH, Kim WS, Cheon JE, et al. Radiological spectrum of hepatic mesenchymal hamartoma in children. Korean J Radiol 2007;8(6):498–505.

28. Lauwers GY, Grant LD, Donnelly WH, et al. Hepatic undifferentiated (embryonal) sarcoma arising in a mesenchymal hamartoma. Am J Surg Pathol 1997;21(10):1248–54.

29. De Chedarevian JP, Pawel BR, Faerber EN, et al. Undifferentiated (embryonal) sarcoma arising in conjunction with mesenchymal hamartoma of the liver. Mod Pathol 1994;7(4):490–3.

30. O'Sullivan MJ, Swanson PE, Knoll J, et al. Undifferentiated embryonal sarcoma with unusual features arising within mesenchymal hamartoma of the liver: report of a case and review of the literature. Pediatr Dev Pathol 2001;4(5):482–9.

31. Li Q, Wang J, Sun Y, et al. Hepatic angiosarcoma arising in an adult mesenchymal hamartoma. Int Semin in Surg Oncol 2007;4:3.

32. Grazioli L, Federle MP, Brancatelli G, et al. Hepatic adenomas: imaging and pathologic findings. Radiographics 2001;21:877–94.

33. Kerlin P, Davis GL, McGill DB, et al. Hepatic adenoma and focal nodular hyperplasia: clinical, pathologic and radiologic features. Gastroenterology 1983;84:994–1002.

34. Brunelle F, Tammam S, Odievre M, et al. Liver adenomas in glycogen storage disease in children. Pediatr Radiol 1984;14:94–101.

35. Beutow PC, Pantongrag-Brown L, Buck JL, et al. From the archives of the AFIP: focal nodular hyperplasia of the liver: radiologic-pathologic correlation. Radiographics 1996;16(2):369–88.

36. Toma P, Taccone A, Martinoli C. MRI of hepatic focal nodular hyperplasia: a report of two new cases in the pediatric age group. Pediatr Radiol 1990;20:267–9.

37. Dachman AH, Pakter RL, Ros PR, et al. Hepatoblastoma: radiologic-pathologic correlation in 50 cases. Radiology 1987;164:15–9.

38. Dubois J, Garel L, Russo P, et al. Pediatric case of the day. Radiographics 1993;13:691–2.

39. Friedman AC, Lichtenstein JE, Goodman Z, et al. Fibrolamellar hepatocellular carcinoma. Radiology 1985;157(3):583–7.

40. Katzenstein H, Krallo MD, Malogolowkin M, et al. Fibrolamellar hepatocellular carcinoma in children and adolescents. Cancer 2003;97:2006–12.

41. Brant DJ, Johnson CD, Stephens DH, et al. Imaging of fibrolamellar hepatocellular carcinoma. AJR Am J Roentgenol 1988;151:295–9.

42. Moon WK, Kim WS, Kim IO, et al. Undifferentiated embryonal sarcoma of the liver: US and CT findings. Pediatr Radiol 1994;24:500–3.

43. McHugh K. Renal and adrenal tumors in children. Cancer Imaging 2007;7:41–51.

44. Miller JH, Greenspan BS. Integrated imaging of hepatic tumors in childhood. Radiology 1985;154:83–90.

45. Leite NP, Kased N, Hanna RF, et al. Cross-sectional imaging of extranodal involvement in abdominopelvic lymphoproliferative malignancies. Radiographics 2007;27:1613–34.

46. Bowen AD, Meza MP, Ledesma-Medina J, et al. Cases of the day: pediatric case of the day. Radiographics 1992;12:393–5.

47. Strouse PJ, Platt JL, Francis IR, et al. Tumorous intrahepatic lymphoproliferative disorder in transplanted livers. AJR Am J Roentgenol 1996;167:1159–62.

New Techniques in Pediatric Ultrasound

Dana Dumitriu, MD[a], Marie-Agnès Galloy, MD[a,b],
Michel Claudon, MD[a,b],*

KEYWORDS

- US • Technology • Doppler modes
- Contrast-enhanced ultrasound • 3D imaging
- Elastography

Ultrasound (US) has been an essential part of pediatric imaging ever since its beginnings because children are the ones who benefit the most from its lack of irradiation and availability. Imaging developing organs and dealing with specific physiologic processes required development of better US probes and adaptation of imaging protocols, leading to a successful contribution to the management of many pediatric diseases. In the last decade, new techniques and modes have brought a further contribution to the ever-expanding applications of US in pediatric pathology.

The objectives of this article are to review the main technical advances that have been recently introduced, to discuss their advantages and limits in children, and to present future perspectives to be considered by the pediatric community.

ADVANCES IN US TECHNOLOGY
From Ceramics to Capacitive Micromachined Ultrasonic Transducers

Research in this field has been extremely active for the last decade. Companies have introduced new piezoelectric materials with lower characteristic acoustic impedances and greater electromechanical coupling coefficients, such as pure wave crystal technique (Philips Bothell, WA, USA). The internal architecture of probes has become more and more complex (ie, associating several layers of elements). Improvements in the control of the way small transducer elements vibrate and in the construction of absorbing backing and matching layers, has been achieved, allowing more accurate profiling of US transmission pulses.[1,2]

The most recent advance is represented by the introduction of capacitive micromachined ultrasonic transducers (CMUTs). The principle is to replace conventional ceramics by small elements made of a nitride membrane vibrating on a silicon wafer, allowing for both the transmission of the US waves and the reception of backscattered echoes (**Fig. 1**). Expected advantages of this new technique include impedance values close to that of soft tissue, increased resolution, better portability of probes, and potentially lower costs of production (Siemens, Erlangen, Germany; Hitachi Medical Japan). In a recent phantom study, CMUT probe was shown to exhibit similar image quality as compared with a state-of-the-art piezocomposite probe, with slightly improved

The authors appreciate the assistance and support of ultrasound manufacturing companies, Esaote, General Electric, Hitachi, Philips, Siemens, Supersonic Imagine, Toshiba, and Zonare.

[a] Department of Radiology, Children's Hospital and INSERM-ERI13, Rue du Morvan, 54511 Vandoeuvre les Nancy, France

[b] University of Nancy, Avenue de la Forêt de Haye, 54511 Vandoeuvre-les-Nancy, France

* Corresponding author. Department of Radiology, Children's Hospital and INSERM-ERI13, Rue du Morvan, 54511 Vandoeuvre les Nancy, France.
E-mail address: m.claudon@chu-nancy.fr

Ultrasound Clin 5 (2010) 153–169
doi:10.1016/j.cult.2009.11.015

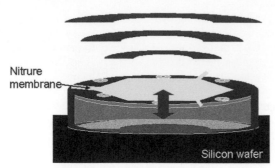

Fig. 1. Diagram of a CMUT. (*Courtesy of* Siemens, Erlangen, Germany; with permission.)

resolution, significantly enhanced contrast, and superior field of view.[3] However, the sensitivity of CMUTs in gray scale and Doppler modes remains to be evaluated in large clinical trials.

Advantages of Broadband Transducers

Bearing in mind that, from a theoretical point of view, the shorter the pulse length, the broader the pulse bandwidth, the main benefit of using a broadband transducer is the improvement of the axial resolution, due to shorter pulse lengths (**Fig. 2**).[2] With broadband transducers, higher transmission frequencies give a better spatial resolution in the near field, whereas lower frequencies allow better penetration in the far field. Very broad bandwidth transducers are now available and, for example, recent linear transducers have frequencies up to 13 or 16 MHz, allowing superior evaluation from very superficial organs to a few centimeters in depth (**Fig. 3**).

Modulating and Associating Pulses

As explained above, the response of piezoelectric materials can be readily tailored, which allows sharp modulation of the pulse characteristics, including the transmission frequency bandwidth, amplitude, phase and length, and the emission of successive pulses. As a relative variable, phase can be determined by comparison with a reference waveform, or with another pulse. Using multiple beamformers allows the direct integration of the phase information from the signal received from adjacent lines (Siemens, Erlangen, Germany).

Currently, a large variety of modulated pulses and pulse sequences have been introduced by most US manufacturers. These processes include single-pulse, multipulse, and multiline techniques. They have greatly contributed to the improvement of imaging quality and the introduction of new US modes, such as harmonic imaging, as illustrated in the following paragraphs.

Spatial Insonation Techniques and Temporal Resolution

In conventional systems working with one beamformer, the information is captured by sending and receiving hundreds of individual "lines" to form an image (**Fig. 4**A). The frame rate is limited by the number of lines of an image the system is able to compute in parallel, with a maximum of approximately 50 to 60 images per second.

By blanketing fewer, larger zones in one shot, large amounts of imaging information can be acquired all at once, with a frame rate going up to 10 times faster than with conventional systems (Zonare Medical Systems, Mountain View, CA, USA) (**Fig. 4**B).

It is also possible to send ultrasound plane or flat waves into tissues to insonify the full imaging plane in one shot, while limiting the acoustic power to safe levels. Then, the maximum frame rate achievable is determined by the time it takes for the US wave to travel from the transducer to the tissue and back. For example, for a 4 cm deep field, the maximum frame rate achievable is

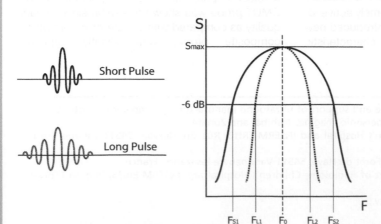

Fig. 2. Broadband transducers. The thresholds are defined by a minus 6dB below the maximum signal. A shorter pulse length gives a broader pulse bandwidth (*dotted line*) compared with a longer one (*plain line*). F_0 mean transmission frequency; F_{L1} and F_{L2}, thresholds of band with for a long pulse; F_{S1} and F_{S2}, thresholds of band with for a short pulse.

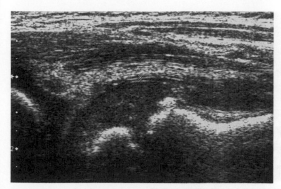

Fig. 3. Musculoskeletal ultrasound with a 5–15 MHz probe, showing superficial and deeper tissues.

approximately 20,000 Hz. The technical challenge is the ability to process the US images acquired at such ultrafast frame rates (Supersonic Imagine, Aix en Provence France) (**Fig. 4**C).

Miniaturization and Portable Machines

New technology is now enabling the miniaturization of high-performance ultrasound equipment capable of performing complete examinations. Handheld ultrasound units—introduced a decade ago[4]—now represent approximately 10% of the market, with a rapidly increasing growth rate. The design, weight, battery life, choice of transducers, capabilities, and modes may vary considerably between units, and it is not the purpose of this article to give an analysis of a moving market. However, the current trend is to have compact but powerful units, allowing radiologists and clinicians to perform high-quality ultrasound in most clinical circumstances, including emergency rooms and ICUs. Very small machines, sometimes called "acoustic stethoscopes," are also promoted by some companies.

Miniaturization is also very active in developing new specialized transducers such as endovascular, laparoscopic, and transesophageal probes.

IMPROVING TWO-DIMENSIONAL GRAYSCALE IMAGE QUALITY
Improving Spatial Resolution

The improvement in piezoelectric materials, the design of transducers, early digitization, and better analysis of received echoes with a lower level of noise allow the use of ever higher transmission frequencies for imaging. This results in higher axial and lateral spatial resolution. For example, it is now possible to evaluate the liver or the kidney in children with linear probes providing more anatomic detail or different echogenicity than

obtained with conventional, lower frequencies probes (**Fig. 5**).

Electronic dynamic focusing at emission and reception is a classical way to improve lateral resolution. In the dynamic transmit focusing modality (Siemens, Erlangen, Germany), edge elements have a longer pulse excitation than center elements, making the US beam focus at two different points in the insonated field, further improving lateral resolution.[5]

Improvement of the elevational resolution is also a challenge for ultrasound imaging. The emerging applications of contrast agent imaging and three-dimensional (3D) require thinner and more uniform image slice thickness for reduction of partial-volume artifacts and better performance. A decade ago, the introduction of so-called 1.5D transducers, which are designed to include three to seven parallel rows of short elements, made some progress in this direction. The method allows focusing control in the z-plane, but requires the management of a high number of channels.[1]

Another approach is to add a special acoustic lens (Hanafy Lens, Siemens, Erlangen, Germany) that uses a variable-thickness crystal to produce a narrow and uniform image slice thickness, and simultaneously an extremely broad bandwidth pulse. The outer portion of the crystal resonates at the lowest frequency, and is focused in both transmission and reception at the deepest part of the image where the low frequencies also provide better penetration. The central portion is thinner, resonates at higher frequencies, and focuses more superficially.[5]

Improving Penetration

With broadband transducers, the use of short pulses results in a high axial resolution, which is beneficial for imaging. However, the lower level of energy transmitted to tissues by such short pulses compromises penetration because of attenuation effects.[6]

There are two main technical solutions to overcome this limitation. In chirped emission (Siemens, Erlangen, Germany), a long, specially shaped transmitter pulse (a chirp) varies in frequency and amplitude within the duration of the pulse itself (**Fig. 6**A). On receive, echoes pass through a filter that is an exact time-reversed replica of the transmitted chirp. As a result, the image has very high axial resolution, increased signal-to-noise ratio, and increased penetration. In coded-emission mode (General Electric Healthcare, Chalfont St Giles, UK; Esaote Biomedica, Genoa, Italy), the scanner does not transmit a single pulse but, instead, a sequence of short,

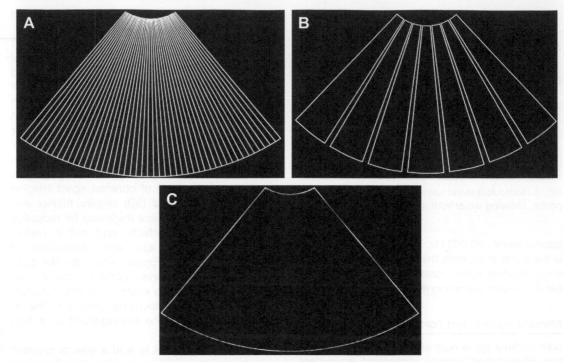

Fig. 4. Spatial insonication techniques. (*A*) Conventional system with insonication by individual lines. (*B*) Sonography with insonication by zone (*Courtesy of* Zonare, Mountain View, CA, USA; with permission), allowing faster frame rates. (*C*) Full-image insonication in one shot, providing very high frame rates. (*Courtesy of* Supersonics Imagine, Aix en Provence, France; with permission.)

high-frequency transmission pulses that may have different phases and are modulated in a code sequence (**Fig. 6**B). Comparison between transmitted pulses and received signal shapes using matched filtering (decoding) is subsequently performed with a very high sampling rate.[7] This second technique, which has long been used in radar and sonar, also results in increasing image penetration without compromising axial resolution or increasing the transmitted peak pressures.

Improving Contrast Resolution

Transmit compounding mode
The principle of compounding, which is now available on most US machines, is to combine images that have been obtained using different spatial angles (**Fig. 7**A).[6] The digital beamformer electronically steers transducer arrays usually from 5 up to 11 steering angles, at real-time acquisition rates. Compounding improves the contrast resolution

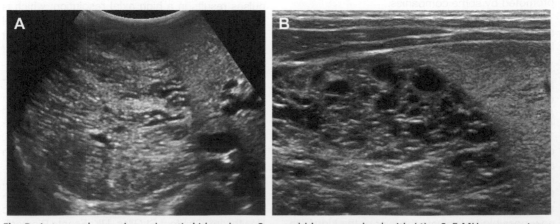

Fig. 5. Autosomal recessive polycystic kidney in an 8-year-old boy, examined with (*A*) a 3–5 MHz convex transducer and (*B*) a 5–12 MHz linear transducer. By examining the renal parenchyma with a high transmission frequencies transducer, the kidney appears less echoic, as small renal cysts are better defined.

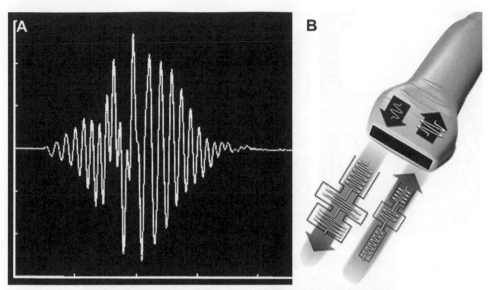

Fig. 6. Solutions to improve penetration. (*A*) Transmitted chirped pulse, which is shaped in amplitude (*Courtesy of* Siemens, Erlangen, Germany; with permission). (*B*) Coded pulse technique transmitting a coded pulse sequence and decoding the pulse sequence on receive with a decoder (*Courtesy of* General Electric Health care, Chalfrant, UK; with permission).

of soft tissues and lesions by reducing artifacts such as speckle, clutter, and noise without compromising other beneficial image characteristics such as spatial resolution. The shadowing from highly reflecting structures is also reduced, which is usually beneficial. But this may be a concern for stones, calcifications or gas, for which the reduction of the posterior acoustic shadowing may be disturbing for the radiologist (**Fig. 7**B,C).

The simultaneous emission of two frequencies transmit frequency compounding (Siemens, Erlangen, Germany) results in better contrast resolution, in addition to the reduction of both noise and speckle.[8]

Nonlinear or harmonic imaging
When US pulses propagate through tissues, their frequency content is altered by numerous mechanisms. The peaks of the pressure waves travel slightly faster than the troughs because of the different velocity of ultrasound propagation in compressed tissue when compared with relaxed tissue, progressively generating harmonics.[9–11] The amplitude of the nonlinear response of tissues is related to the nonlinear parameter B/A, which is an inherent characteristic of the tissue.[12]

Tissue harmonic imaging (THI) is based on the exploitation of the harmonics generated by this nonlinear response of tissues. Currently, most ultrasound devices use the second harmonic (twice the initial frequency), since exploiting higher harmonic frequencies would require very broad

bandwidth transducers.[5,13] THI requires the suppression of the fundamental component of the backscattered signal, which is of a higher intensity than the harmonic one. This has been first achieved by simply using receive filters to filter out the pure fundamental signal, allowing the image then to be reconstructed from the remaining harmonic signal.[14] Currently, the generally preferred method is to use multipulse techniques, mainly the pulse phase inversion sequences in which two pulses of opposite polarity are transmitted along the same line. The subtraction process of the two signals results in a relative increase in signal from tissue nonlinear response by canceling the linear component (**Fig. 8**).

Among the advantages of THI are better axial and lateral resolution, and the reduction of artifacts such as side lobes and scattering.[5] THI has been found to be useful in obese patients, where the abdominal wall produces beam attenuation and defocusing; this does not happen as much in THI because the harmonic waves are produced inside the tissue and not at the surface of the ultrasound transducer, which reduces the artifacts of the abdominal wall to a certain degree.[13] Although the issue of overweight children posing the same problems for ultrasound as adults is more and more present in day-to-day practice, it is certain that there are also other benefits to THI.

It has been assessed that THI enhances "good" artifacts (shadow artifact) and reduces "bad" artifacts (lobe, ring-down, and volume averaging).[6]

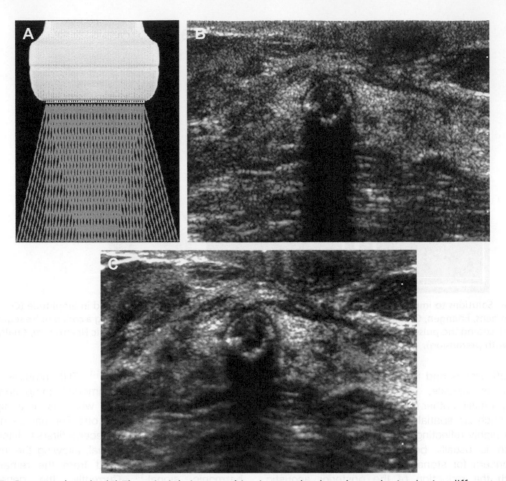

Fig. 7. Compound mode. (*A*) The principle is to combine images that have been obtained using different spatial orientations. (*Courtesy of* Philips, Bothell, USA; with permission.) (*B*) Large posterior acoustic shadowing observed behind a fecalith on baseline mode. (*C*) Marked reduction of the posterior shadowing by applying the compounding mode.

Lesion definition and contrast, differential diagnosis between small cystic, and solid nodules are improved, sometimes at the price of a certain loss of penetration.[15] Structures containing air, such as the digestive tract, calcifications, or other highly reflective tissues, also benefit from THI.[13] In acute appendicitis, THI allows a better visualization of the appendiceal wall and contents and a better appreciation of the adjacent inflamed mesentery and of the bowel loops.[16] The improved assessment of the digestive tract has also been described for inflammatory bowel diseases, which represent another important pathology in the adolescent age group.[17]

THI applications have also been recently described in the evaluation of the urinary tract.[18] Darge and Heidemeier[19] found that THI was superior to conventional (fundamental) ultrasound imaging in the depiction of several parameters such as: visualization of the bladder wall and retrovesical space, renal contrast to liver or spleen,

the pelvicalyceal systems, and corticomedullary differentiation. This was statistically significant for the dorsal approach for all parameters, whereas for the ventral approach, THI was useful especially for a better visualization of the bladder wall and the pelvicalyceal system (**Fig. 9**).[18] THI has already found some place in echocardiography, where it seems to be superior to conventional ultrasound in imaging children with poor acoustic windows.[19]

Finally, it is possible to combine compounding and THI to further improve image quality (**Fig. 10A–D**).

MOVING BEYOND TWO-DIMENSIONAL IMAGING
Extended-field Acquisition

Extended field-of-view sonography has now been included in most machines, generally for both grayscale and power Doppler modes. The

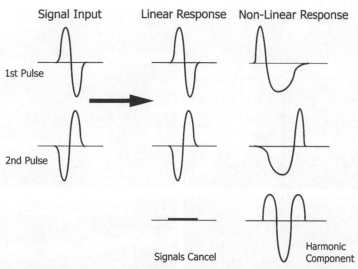

Fig. 8. Principle of pulse inversion. Two pulses of opposite polarity are transmitted along the same line. The subtraction process results in cancellation of the linear component of the signal and a relative increase in the nonlinear response from tissues.

information regarding position is recovered directly from the ultrasound images themselves, allowing the reconstruction of a wide image by a progressive addition of data acquired during a hand sweep. Extended field-of-view has been demonstrated to allow measurement of large structures and reveal the anatomic context of abnormalities in circumstances under which conventional real-time scans could not provide the information.[20]

3D Imaging

The principle of volume ultrasound (3DUS) is the combination of a two-dimensional (2D) acquisition and positional information, which permits the

reconstruction of a volume.[21] Chronologically, several types of 3D acquisitions have been developed:

1. Freehand scanning, initially without a position sensor, then combined with an electromagnetic, optical, or mechanic position sensor.
2. Mechanic 3D transducers, which are rather large systems, as they contain a motor to tilt a conventional 2D probe typically ranging between 20 and 75 degrees. The in-plane spatial resolution of the 3D acquisition is first determined by the resolution of the 2D probe, whereas the resolution in other planes is lower, depending on the depth and obliquity of the plane.

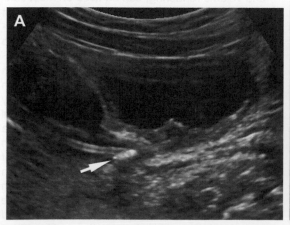
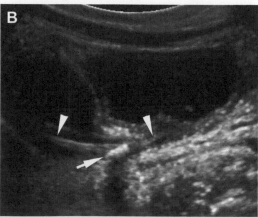

Fig. 9. Lithiasis in a pelvic ureter in a young boy. (A) The stone (arrow) is hardly seen on the fundamental mode image. (B) The stone (arrow) with its posterior acoustic shadowing and the ureteral stent (arrowheads) are better displayed on harmonic mode images.

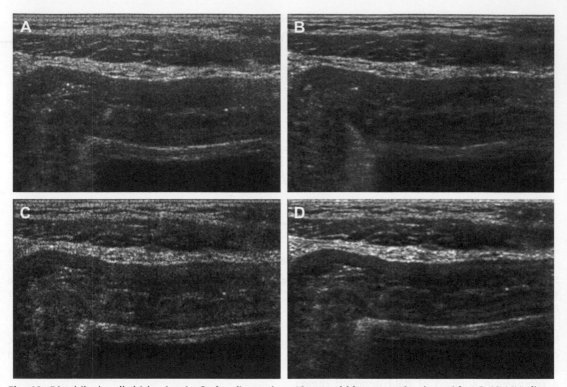

Fig. 10. Distal ileal wall thickening in Crohn disease in a 10-year-old boy; examination with a 5–12 MHz linear transducer. (*A*) Fundamental image. (*B*) Compound mode. (*C*) THI mode. (*D*) Compound plus THI mode. Compounding mode allows better visualization of the bowel layers. By adding harmonic imaging, the layers of the bowel wall are also better defined, but the artifacts from the abdominal wall are enhanced as well. Combining THI and compound modes produces the best image, with a good definition of the bowel wall and reduction of artifacts.

3. Matrix transducers containing approximately 2,500 to 9,000 elements acquire volumetric data by a complex, phased-array sweep across the pyramid-shaped volume. The resolution depends on the number of elements of the matrix, but, as for any phased-array transducer, currently remains below the one provided by mechanic probes. The two main advantages for this type of transducer are the small size, which makes them easier to use in children, and a much higher temporal resolution.

4. Four-dimensional US is obtained by consecutive fast updates of the 3D data set, allowing a dynamic 3D visualization of the volume. Frame rates obtained with matrix probes are higher compared with mechanical probes.

Having a good quality 3D volume depends primarily on having a proper 2D examination: the same artifacts will intervene for 3D US as for conventional US, and areas which are difficult to examine with conventional ultrasound will be problematic for the 3D acquisition as well.[22] Once acquired, the volume may be analyzed entirely in any number of planes. It may be rendered as a single slice of a chosen thickness or as an entire volume. The main post-processing tools like multiplanar reconstruction, maximum intensity projection, minimum intensity projection, and volume rendering, can be used on most software and workstations to improve the quality of the image display in order to better reveal the suspected pathology or demonstrate its relationship with surrounding structures (**Fig. 11**).

Although it has become a common tool in obstetric ultrasound, the clinical experience with body 3D US in the pediatric population has only be recently initiated. There are several potential limitations in children. First, the maximum value of the acquisition angle is currently 75°, which may be insufficient to cover the entire region of interest, such as a large tumor. Second, when using mechanical transducers, the acquisition time is proportional to the angle chosen by the examiner and may be too long for a small child to obtain a volume free from motion and breathing artifacts. This problem may, however, be greatly reduced by the development of the matrix

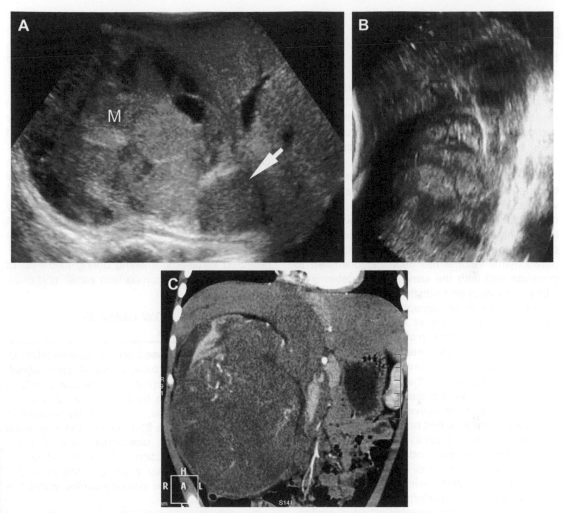

Fig. 11. Right nephroblastoma in a 1-year-old boy. (*A*) 2D images reveal a large renal mass (M) with venous extension to the renal vein and the inferior vena cava (*arrow*). (*B*) 3D coronal multiplanar reconstruction image displays the tumor and the complete venous extension. (*C*) CT correlation in a coronal view.

transducers, the acquisition time being much shorter.[23] Third, the resolution of the images in the reconstructed planes remains generally inferior to that of a 2D acquisition, which may cause difficulties in identifying subtle parenchymal changes or small focal lesions.[24] Nevertheless, the image quality should benefit from the introduction of higher frequency transducers, improving both spatial and contrast resolution.

3D acquisitions of the neonatal brain have been achieved, correctly demonstrating the normal anatomy and allowing the reconstruction of the standard ultrasound coronal and sagittal slices and the visualization of anomalies in any plane.[24] In the neonatal population, it has been demonstrated that 3D ultrasound correctly identifies the presence, location, and extent of hemorrhage,[25] and of lesions such as cysts, tumors, and territorial

infarction.[26] Another important application may be the correct measurement of ventricular volume, especially in the follow-up of hydrocephalus: 3D ultrasound offers an accurate measurement of the normal or dilated ventricles, which is harder to obtain with 2D ultrasound because of irregular ventricular shape.[27] The correlation between the ventricular volume measured by 3D ultrasound and MR imaging has already been demonstrated.[27] Thus, 3D ultrasound volume measurement may become a tool in the detection of subtle developmental anomalies at birth, revealing themselves initially only by an abnormal ventricular volume and for the evaluation and follow-up of hydrocephalus.[28]

Since renal pathology is very common in the pediatric population, 3D ultrasound has already been evaluated in terms of measurement accuracy, and, to a lesser degree in terms of diagnostic abilities. Common day-to-day measurements of the kidneys, dilated cavities, and bladder with 2D ultrasound are not accurate enough. In vitro studies (on animal or synthetic kidney models) and studies comparing ultrasound measurements with MR imaging and CT volume measurements have demonstrated that computing the values measured by 2D ultrasound using the ellipsoid formula produces an error of 15% to 25%.[23,29,30]

With 3D ultrasound, the renal parenchymal volume can be calculated by subtracting the volume of the dilated cavities from the total renal volume.[24] It also may now be directly calculated using a manual segmentation on serial slices covering the organ (**Fig. 12**). The calculated renal parenchymal volume has been demonstrated to correlate well with the same volume determined with MR imaging and with the renal volume determined by renal scintigraphy.[30] Therefore, 3D ultrasound surveillance of children with hydronephrosis, with estimation of the renal and dilated cavity volume, may become a regular application of ultrasound in infant renal pathology, without subjecting the patient to the irradiation of scintigraphy or to a long and costly examination such as MR imaging. Moreover, 3D ultrasound is a useful tool in depicting complex anatomic relationships that may occur in congenital malformations or focal lesions, and in helping to better visualize and differentiate cystic lesions from diverticula or dilated cavities.[22,30] The surface-rendering mode of the volume analysis is regarded as a potential tool for obtaining a "virtual cystoscopy" view of the inner surface of the bladder wall and for identifying abnormalities in the position of the ureteral ostia and congenital anomalies such as ureterocele (**Fig. 13**).[22]

3D US may also be coupled with color Doppler ultrasound or power Doppler, which improves the characterization of focal lesions (such as areas of pyelonephritis, renal infarct, renal trauma, and solid tumors) (**Fig. 14**).[24]

Finally, the introduction of volumetric US protocols in a department is likely to induce changes in the workflow, as the scanning time spent with the patient is reduced, but more time may be needed to analyze the volume in all the desired planes. Conversely, a better efficiency has been shown in prenatal imaging, based on a standardized acquisition of five volumes covering the fetus.[31] An expected advantage of 3D US is the possibility to repeat the analysis of a given region of interest or to share it with different readers without the need to re-examine the patient. In addition, repeated volumetric imaging during follow-up of a lesion may make comparison easier and more reliable.

IMPROVING US FLOW IMAGING
Doppler Techniques

Power Doppler is based on the quantification of the power (the amplitude) of the Doppler signal. There is a loss of information on the flow direction, but the sensitivity to flow is increased and the dependence on angle minimized. By separating positive and negative flows before the estimation of the signal power, directional power Doppler allows the flow direction to be encoded in real time with a two-color scale but still does not provide any detail on hemodynamics within the vessel.[5]

Dynamic Flow (Toshiba, Tokyo, Japan) is based on a broadband Doppler technique, using much shorter pulses than conventional Doppler imaging. Therefore, the spatial resolution of the Doppler map is improved, similar to B-mode grayscale

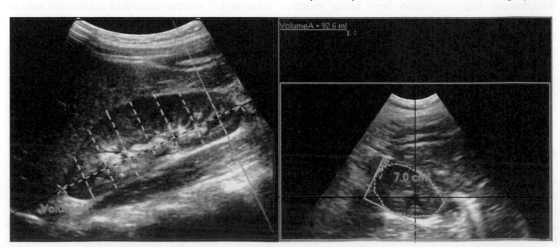

Fig. 12. Calculating the renal volume by the stacked ellipses method (3D mode, Philips, Bothell, USA).

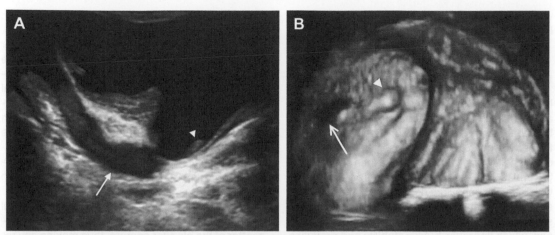

Fig. 13. 3D ultrasound of the bladder in a 15-year-old patient treated for vesicoureteral reflux by the injection of dextranomer/hyaluronic acid copolymer (Deflux). (*A*) The thick-slice rendering of the acquired volume reveals an incorrect position of the antireflux material (*arrowhead*) with persistent dilatation of the ureter (*arrow*). (*B*) Virtual cystoscopy rendering of the same volume demonstrates the contour of the antireflux material (*arrowhead*) and the ostium of the dilated ureter (*arrow*).

imaging. However, because of a lower energy level delivered to tissues and attenuation effects, the sensitivity may be lower for deep and slow-flow vessels.

Graycale Flow-imaging Techniques

Graycale flow-imaging techniques are based on B-mode and allow the simultaneous imaging of blood flow and tissues without a threshold decision and color overlay, which is usually necessary in Doppler modes. B-flow (General Electric Healthcare, Chalfont St Giles, UK) works by comparing the backscattered signals from a pair of coded pulse sequences emitted with a very short time gap. If blood cells have moved between the two pulses, then the two received signals will be slightly different, and if they are subtracted one from another, there will not be perfect cancellation. The remaining signal can then be boosted and displayed as a representation of movement. Signal brightness is determined by blood echo strength and blood

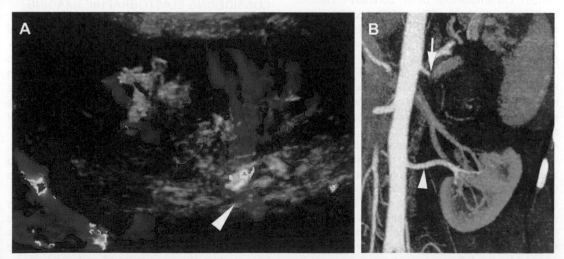

Fig. 14. Traumatic dissection of the main artery of the left kidney in a 15-year-old girl. (*A*) 3D Doppler ultrasound shows the absence of vessels in the upper and middle pole of the kidney, and a patent inferior polar artery (*arrowhead*). (*B*) CT correlation confirms the proximal dissection of the main artery (*arrow*) and normal flow within the inferior accessory artery (*arrowhead*).

velocity but it is not a linear relationship.[5,32] There is little application in pediatrics published to date.

INTRODUCING CEUS IN PEDIATRIC IMAGING

Ultrasound contrast agents (UCAs) are blood-pool agents, which allow the assessment of blood flow by enhancing the ultrasound backscatter. They are formed of microbubbles of gas, stabilized by an outer shell, with a diameter of less than 5 microns.[33] Several UCAs are currently marketed worldwide, with different behaviors depending on their composition. The most currently used agents are so-called second-generation UCAs made of low-solubility gas, which improves bubble stability and produces favorable resonance behavior at low acoustic pressure. This allows minimally disruptive imaging and enables effective investigations over several minutes with the visualization of the dynamic enhancement pattern in real time.[33] Specific modes, such as contrast-specific harmonic imaging or phase inversion imaging are required to adequately display the signal from the microbubbles, and several protocols have been described.[33] UCAs are safer than iodine-based conventional contrast material and they are not nephrotoxic. The rate of severe allergic reactions to ultrasound contrast agents is very low, with a reported incidence of 0.001% in abdominal usage in adult populations.[34]

Although less research has been done to characterize the performance of contrast-enhanced ultrasound (CEUS) in the pediatric population, pediatric radiologists should pay attention to this ultrasound application, as it might replace in certain circumstances other contrast-enhanced techniques such as CT or MR imaging, thus reducing radiation exposure and costs. However, most agents have not been yet approved for pediatric use.

Based on a limited personal experience, characterization of focal liver lesions in children appear similar with the adult population: in the portal-late phase, sustained enhancement characterizes most benign solid liver lesions (**Fig. 15**), while hypoenhancement mainly characterizes malignancies.[35]

CEUS has been evaluated in the context of pediatric blunt abdominal trauma and found to improve the detection of solid organ lesions by comparison to unenhanced ultrasound, especially in equivocal cases where free peritoneal fluid was not present (**Fig. 16**).[36] Using two boluses of contrast material, one to examine the right upper quadrant and the second for the left upper quadrant, the sensitivity of ultrasound was 92.9%, with a specificity of 100%, compared with contrast-enhanced abdominal CT.[36] The difficulties in identifying diaphragmatic, bowel, or mesenteric traumatic lesions are limitations of CEUS.[36]

Probably the most researched application for CEUS in the pediatric population has been the exploration of vesicoureteral reflux by voiding urosonography, in the attempt to replace traditional voiding cystourethrography (VCUG) and radionuclide cystography. Several studies have shown that voiding urosonography could be a reliable and feasible examination. Levovist (Schering, Berlin, Germany) is the only agent approved for intracavitary administration in several European countries.

When instilled in the bladder via a transurethral catheter, the UCA greatly enhances the backscatter of the bladder content, thus making any reflux within the ureters or the pelvicalyceal system more visible.[37] The sensitivity of VUS for detecting small vesicoureteral reflux using Levovist seems to be greater than that of VCUG.[38] A few studies have been published using Sonovue (Bracco, Milano, Italy), also indicating excellent sensitivity (**Fig. 17**).[39]

Some centers use a complement of transperineal CEUS of the urethra with pre-, intra-, and postvoiding examination of the posterior urethra, to detect posterior urethral valves,[40] but it may be difficult to evaluate both the urethra and upper urinary tract at the same time, during voiding.

Because of all these considerations, VUS is preferred as a follow-up alternative to VCUG for boys, but it has become the initial examination for girls in some centers.[33,37]

CONSIDERING ELASTOGRAPHIC IMAGING

Palpation is an important component of the clinical examination in any age group. Achieving a quantification of the information provided by palpation is the goal of elastography. Its principle lies in applying external pressure to a structure or tissue and measuring the relative displacement of the reflective target, thus determining the degree of deformability or elasticity of a given structure.[41] Using cross-correlation methods to determine the position of reflective structures before and after compression, elastography creates a map of the tension profile in a given tissue.

To determine the tension profile and thus the elasticity pattern in a region of interest, real-time elastography receives the radiofrequency waves produced by the reflected ultrasound wave in the tissues, thus obtaining a line of an A-mode sonogram, and measures the displacement of the radiofrequency source before and after compression. To obtain a bidimensional elastogram, the

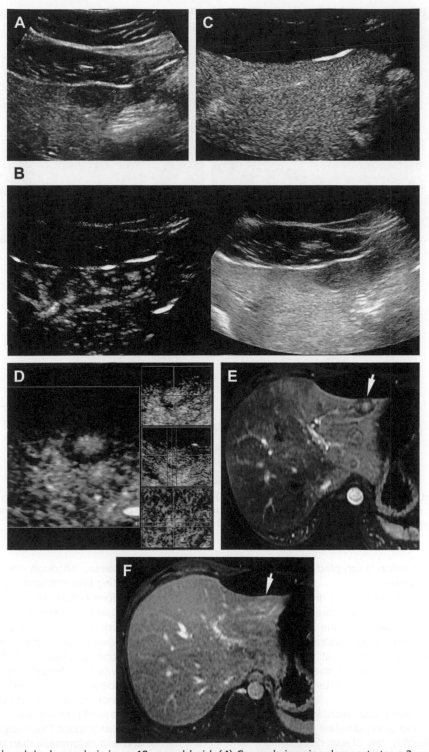

Fig. 15. Focal nodular hyperplasia in an 18-year-old girl. (*A*) Grayscale imaging demonstrates a 2 cm hypoechoic nodule of the left hepatic lobe. (*B*) Dual screen CEUS obtained 10 seconds after the intravenous administration of a bolus of 2.4 mL of Sonovue (*Courtesy of* Bracco, Milano, Italy; with permission) shows bubbles starting to fill the lesion from the center. (*C*) Sustained enhancement is observed during the portal and late phases. (*D*) 3D contrast-enhanced sonography during the arterial phase better shows the centrifugal filling of the lesion. Contrast-enhanced MR images obtained during the (*E*) arterial and (*F*) portal phases correlate well with the CEUS images (*arrow points to lesion*).

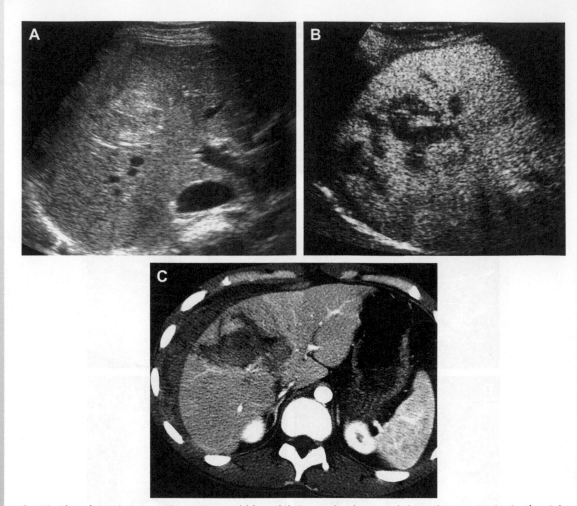

Fig. 16. Blunt hepatic trauma in a 15-year-old boy. (*A*) Grayscale ultrasound shows heterogeneity in the right hepatic lobe. (*B*) Contrast-enhanced imaging precisely demonstrates the presence of several fracture lines within the parenchyma and the capsule at the dome level. (*C*) Contrast-enhanced CT correlation.

elasticity information is sampled on several longitudinal parallel axes.[41]

Developed specifically for liver applications, transient elastography is a different method, which uses a vibrator attached to the ultrasound probe and induces low-frequency vibrations transmitted through the tissue. Tissue stiffness is directly proportional to the square of shear wave velocity: the stiffer the tissue, the faster the shear wave propagates.

In the shear wave approach, focusing the ultrasonic beam and using ultrafast imaging allow to precisely quantify the shear displacement with the expectation of a higher spatial resolution and less artifacts than with conventional elastography method (Supersonic Imagine, Aix en Provence, France).

In liver pathology, transient and real-time elastography have been widely evaluated in adults in

diffuse liver disease. Although the benefits of correctly estimating liver stiffness and quantifying the degree of fibrosis without reverting to liver biopsy are particularly interesting in children, there are few studies oriented toward the pediatric population. Liver studies have focused mostly on transient elastography (Fibroscan, Echosens SA, Paris, France), which is feasible in children[42,43] and correctly identifies advanced degrees of fibrosis, but cannot distinguish between stages 1 and 2 in mild cases of liver fibrosis.[43]

Based on the assumption that malignant lesions are harder and less deformable than benign ones, real-time ultrasound elastography already has certain established applications in adult pathology, in particular in breast imaging[44] and for the characterization of focal thyroid nodules.[45]

Although it is still in the early phases of evaluation, real-time elastography could also be a useful

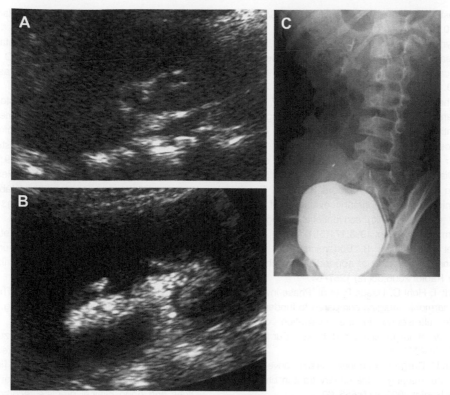

Fig. 17. Right vesicoureteral reflux in a 4-year-old girl. (*A*) Low mechanical index evaluation of the right kidney at baseline. (*B*) After the administration of the contrast (0.5 mL) showing a grade 2 reflux. (*Courtesy of* Sonovue, Bracco, Milano, Italy; with permission.) (*C*) Correlation with retrograde cystography.

tool in pediatric neuromuscular diseases or after orthopedic interventions to determine the structure and contraction characteristics of skeletal muscle.[46] In postoperative circumstances, it has been tested as a tool to determine the effectiveness of muscle reconstruction after cleft lip[47] and anterior cruciate ligament repair.[48]

SUMMARY

The various developments of ultrasound techniques and methods are finding their place in the pediatric radiologist's day-to-day practice, greatly improving and enlarging the applications of this safe and universally available method that is ultrasound. Its lack of radiation exposure and moderate cost should be, in the future, strong arguments toward maintaining it as much as possible as a main imaging technique in the pediatric population.

REFERENCES

1. Rizzatto G. Evolution of ultrasound transducers: 1.5 and 2D arrays. Eur Radiol 1999;9(Suppl 3):S304–6.
2. Whittingham TA. Broadband transducers. Eur Radiol 1999;9(Suppl 3):S298–303.
3. Legros M, Meynier C, Dufait R, et al. Piezocomposite and CMUT arrays assessment through in vitro imaging performances. 2008 IEEE International Ultrasonics Symposium (IUS) Beijing, November 2–5, 2008.
4. Lowers J. Abdominal ultrasound: new technologies alleviate the daily grind. Diagn Imaging 2000;22:63–6.
5. Claudon M, Tranquart F, Evans DH, et al. Advances in ultrasound. Eur Radiol 2002;12(1):7–18.
6. O'Brien RT, Holmes SP. Recent advances in ultrasound technology. Clin Tech Small Anim Pract 2007;22(3):93–103.
7. Chiao R, Mo L, Hall A, et al. B-mode blood flow (B-flow) imaging. In IEEE International Ultrasonics Symposium. Puerto Ricco, October 22–25, 2000.
8. Whittingham TA. Tissue harmonic imaging. Eur Radiol 1999;9(Suppl 3):S323–6.
9. Law W, Frizzell L, Dunn F. Determination of the nonlinearity parameter B/A of biological media. Ultrasound Med Biol 1985;11:307–18.
10. Sehgal C, Brown G, Bahn R, et al. Measurement and use of acoustic nonlinearity and sound speed to estimate composition of excised livers. Ultrasound Med Biol 1986;12:865–74.
11. Ward B, Baker A, Humphrey V. Nonlinear propagation applied to the improvement of resolution in

diagnostic medical ultrasound. J Acoust Soc Am 1997;101:143–54.

12. Filipczynski L, Kujawska T, Tymkiewiwz R, et al. Nonlinear and linear propagation of diagnostic ultrasound pulses. Ultrasound Med Biol 1999;25: 285–99.

13. Choudhry S, Gorman B, Charboneau JW, et al. Comparison of tissue harmonic imaging with conventional US in abdominal disease. Radiographics 2000;20(4):1127–35.

14. Freiherr G. 3-D ultrasound: will it become a clinical tool? Diagn Imaging (San Franc) 1998;20(7):52–7.

15. Shapiro RS, Wagreich J, Parsons RB, et al. Tissue harmonic imaging sonography: evaluation of image quality compared with conventional sonography. AJR Am J Roentgenol 1998;171(5):1203–6.

16. Rompel O, Huelsse B, Bodenschatz K, et al. Harmonic US imaging of appendicitis in children. Pediatr Radiol 2006;36(12):1257–64.

17. Schmidt T, Hohl C, Haage P, et al. Phase-inversion tissue harmonic imaging compared to fundamental B-mode ultrasound in the evaluation of the pathology of large and small bowel. Eur Radiol 2005;15(9):2021–30.

18. Bartram U, Darge K. Harmonic versus conventional ultrasound imaging of the urinary tract in children. Pediatr Radiol 2005;35(7):655–60.

19. Darge K, Heidemeier A. Moderne Ultraschalltechniken und ihre Anwendungen am kindlichen Harntrakt [Modern ultrasound technologies and their application in pediatric urinary tract imaging]. Radiologe 2005;45(12):1101–11 [in German].

20. Sauerbrei EE. Extended field-of-view sonography: utility in clinical practice. J Ultrasound Med 1999; 18(5):335–41.

21. Riccabona M. Modern pediatric ultrasound: potential applications and clinical significance [review]. Clin Imaging 2006;30(2):77–86.

22. Riccabona M, Fritz G, Ring E. Potential applications of three-dimensional ultrasound in the pediatric urinary tract: pictorial demonstration based on preliminary results. Eur Radiol 2003;13(12): 2680–7.

23. Kim HC, Yang DM, Lee SH, et al. Usefulness of renal volume measurements obtained by a 3-dimensional sonographic transducer with matrix electronic arrays. J Ultrasound Med 2008;27(12): 1673–81.

24. Riccabona M. Pediatric three-dimensional ultrasound: basics and potential clinical value. Clin Imaging 2005;29(1):1–5.

25. Salerno CC, Pretorius DH, Hilton SW, et al. Three-dimensional ultrasonographic imaging of the neonatal brain in high-risk neonates: preliminary study. J Ultrasound Med 2000;19(8):549–55.

26. Riccabona M, Nelson TR, Weitzer C, et al. Potential of three-dimensional ultrasound in neonatal and paediatric neurosonography. Eur Radiol 2003; 13(9):2082–93.

27. Gilmore JH, Gerig G, Specter B, et al. Infant cerebral ventricle volume: a comparison of 3-D ultrasound and magnetic resonance imaging. Ultrasound Med Biol 2001;27(8):1143–6.

28. Csutak R, Unterassinger L, Rohrmeister C, et al. Three-dimensional volume measurement of the lateral ventricles in preterm and term infants: evaluation of a standardised computer-assisted method in vivo. Pediatr Radiol 2003;33(2):104–9.

29. Bakker J, Olree M, Kaatee R, et al. Renal volume measurements: accuracy and repeatability of US compared with that of MR imaging. Radiology 1999;211(3):623–8.

30. Riccabona M, Fritz GA, Schollnast H, et al. Hydronephrotic kidney: pediatric three-dimensional US for relative renal size assessment—initial experience. Radiology 2005;236(1):276–83.

31. Benacerraf BR, Shipp TD, Bromley B. Three-dimensional US of the fetus: volume imaging. Radiology 2006;238(3):988–96.

32. Weskott HP. B-flow–eine neue methode zur Blutflussdetektion [B-flow–a new method for detecting blood flow]. Ultraschall Med 2000;21(2):59–65 [in German].

33. Claudon M, Cosgrove D, Albrecht T, et al. Guidelines and good clinical practice recommendations for contrast enhanced ultrasound (CEUS)—update 2008. Ultraschall Med 2008;29(1):28–44.

34. Mandry D, Bressenot A, Galloy MA, et al. Contrast-enhanced ultrasound in fibro-lamellar hepatocellular carcinoma: a case report. Ultraschall Med 2007; 28(6):547–52.

35. Valentino M, Serra C, Pavlica P, et al. Blunt abdominal trauma: diagnostic performance of contrast-enhanced US in children—initial experience. Radiology 2008; 246(3):903–9.

36. Darge K. Diagnosis of vesicoureteral reflux with ultrasonography. Pediatr Nephrol 2002;17(1):52–60.

37. Berrocal T, Gaya F, Arjonilla A, et al. Vesicoureteral reflux: diagnosis and grading with echo-enhanced cystosonography versus voiding cystourethrography. Radiology 2001;221(2):359–65.

38. Mate A, Bargiela A, Mosteiro S, et al. Contrast ultrasound of the urethra in children. Eur Radiol 2003; 13(7):1534–7.

39. Ophir J, Cespedes I, Ponnekanti H, et al. Elastography: a quantitative method for imaging the elasticity of biological tissues. Ultrason Imaging 1991;13(2):111–34.

40. de Ledinghen V, Le Bail B, Rebouissoux L, et al. Liver stiffness measurement in children using FibroScan: feasibility study and comparison with Fibrotest, aspartate transaminase to platelets ratio index, and liver biopsy. J Pediatr Gastroenterol Nutr 2007; 45(4):443–50.

41. Nobili V, Vizzutti F, Arena U, et al. Accuracy and reproducibility of transient elastography for the

diagnosis of fibrosis in pediatric nonalcoholic steato-hepatitis. Hepatology 2008;48(2):442–8.

42. Itoh A, Ueno E, Tohno E, et al. Breast disease: clinical application of US elastography for diagnosis. Radiology 2006;239(2):341–50.

43. Lyshchik A, Higashi T, Asato R, et al. Thyroid gland tumor diagnosis at US elastography. Radiology 2005;237(1):202–11.

44. Rago T, Santini F, Scutari M, et al. Elastography: new developments in ultrasound for predicting malignancy in thyroid nodules. J Clin Endocrinol Metab 2007; 92(8):2917–22.

45. Hong Y, Liu X, Li Z, et al. Real-time ultrasound elastography in the differential diagnosis of benign and malignant thyroid nodules. J Ultrasound Med 2009; 28(7):861–7.

46. Hoyt K, Kneezel T, Castaneda B, et al. Quantitative sonoelastography for the in vivo assessment of skeletal muscle viscoelasticity. Phys Med Biol 2008; 53(15):4063–80.

47. de Korte C, Van Hess N, Lopata R, et al. Quantitative assessment of oral orbicular muscle deformation after cleft lip reconstruction: an ultrasound elastography study. IEEE Trans Med Imaging 2009;28(8):2001–10.

48. Spalazzi JP, Gallina J, Fung-Kee-Fung SD, et al. Elastographic imaging of strain distribution in the anterior cruciate ligament and at the ligament-bone insertions. J Orthop Res 2006;24(10):2001–10.

Diagnosis of fibrosis in pediatric nonalcoholic steato-
hepatitis. Hepatology 2008;48(2):442–8.

42. Itoh A, Ueno E, Tohno E, et al. Breast disease: clinical application of US elastography for diagnosis.
Radiology 2006;239(2):341–50.

43. Lyshchik A, Higashi T, Asato R, et al. Thyroid gland
tumor diagnosis at US elastography. Radiology
2005;237(1):202–11.

44. Rago T, Santini F, Scutari M, et al. Elastography: new
developments in ultrasound for predicting malignancy
in thyroid nodules. J Clin Endocrinol Metab 2007;
92(8):2917–22.

45. Hong Y, Liu X, Li Z, et al. Real-time ultrasound elastography in the differential diagnosis of benign and

malignant thyroid nodules. J Ultrasound Med 2009;
28(7):861–7.

46. Hoyt K, Kneezel T, Castaneda B, et al. Quantitative
sonoelastography for the in vivo assessment of skeletal muscle viscoelasticity. Phys Med Biol 2008;
53(15):4063–80.

47. de Korte CL, van Cleef M, Lopata R, et al. Quantitative
assessment of oral orbicular muscle deformation after
cleft lip reconstruction: an ultrasound elastography
study. IEEE Trans Med Imaging 2009;28(8):2001–10.

48. Spalazzi JP, Gallina J, Fung-Kee-Fung SD, et al.
Elastographic imaging of strain distribution in the
anterior cruciate ligament and at the ligament-bone
insertions. J Orthop Res 2006;24(10):2001–10.

Index

Note: Page numbers of article titles are in **boldface** type.

Ultrasound Clin 5 (2010) 171–175
doi:10.1016/S1556-858X(10)00073-3
1556-858X/10/$ – see front matter © 2010 Elsevier Inc. All rights reserved.